UNDERSTANDING GROWTH HORMONE

UNDERSTANDING GROWTH HORMONE

*New Discoveries to Help Very
Short Children...
Are They Also a Fountain of Youth?*

Neil Shulman, M.D.
Letitia Sweitzer

HIPPOCRENE BOOKS
New York

For information, address:
HIPPOCRENE BOOKS, INC.
171 Madison Avenue
New York NY 10016

Library of Congress Cataloging-in-Publication Data
Shulman, Neil.
    Understanding growth hormone : new discoveries to help very short children : are they also a fountain of youth? / Neil Shulman, Letitia Sweitzer.
        p.   cm.
Includes bibliographic references.
ISBN 0-7818-0071-4
1. Somatotropin—Popular works.   I. Sweitzer, Letitia.
II. Title.
QP572.S6S5   1993   92-21485
612.6'5—dc20   CIP

Printed in the United States of America.

DEDICATION

To my family: John; Chris, Patricia, and Owen; Scott, Helen, and Wilson.
—Letitia Sweitzer

To my family, named (in deference to the subject of this book) in order of height, the shortest first: Mary, Bonnie, Sonnie, Roberta, Andy, Stan, Jonathan, and Larry.
—Neil Shulman

Acknowledgments

Our heartfelt thanks to the physicians and researchers who personally shared their knowledge with us: Stephen W. Anderson, M.D.; James H. Christy, M.D.; R. David Cole, Ph.D.; Floyd L. Culler, M.D.; Joseph M. Kincade, Ph.D.; Lillian R. Meacham, M.D.; John S. Parks, M.D., Ph.D.; Janakiraman Ramashandran, Ph.D.; James Reed, M.D.; Ron G. Rosenfeld, M.D.; Daniel Rudman, M.D.; Robert M. Schultz, M.D.; Michael O. Thorner, M.D.; and Harald Waago, M.D.

We are also very grateful for the personal and professional support of Susan M. Dupuy, Kim Frye, Jenny Stone Humphries, Josephine Jamison, John Jones, Pam Kaplan, Beth Mahaffey, Robin Mahaffey, Kristen Mehrhof, Diane Minick, Nancy Murphy, Holly Palmer Rhodes, Cindy Robertson, Leslee Sinclair, Lisa Thomassen, and Lynn Walker.

We especially want to thank all the patients and families who told us their stories and wish them many more years of health and as many inches of growth as they desire.

We also wish to thank those who gave us permission to use previously published figures to illustrate our text. We are expecially grateful to Nathan McKnight for his lively, original drawings.

And finally, many thanks to the folks at Hippocrene Books, especially our editor Jacek Galazka.

CONTENTS

I. Shot o' Youth, Streak o' Lean — 9

II. Dem 'Mones, Dem 'Mones, Dem Hormones: A Very Short Course in Endocrinology — 21

III. Hurried Hormone History — 35

IV. Growth Hormone — 53

V. Too Much of a Good Thing — 73

VI. Tom Thumb and Other Short Stories — 105

VII. Kids, Growth, and GH — 117

VIII. Brent's Story — 143

IX. GH for More Short Kids? — 165

X. Finding the Short Kids — 199

XI. From Clone to Clinic: The Drug Companies — 215

XII. GH and Adults: Antidote to Aging, Boon to Fertility and Healing? — 225

XIII. GH and the Jock — 251

FINALE: A Parting Toast — 267

References — 269

Index — 287

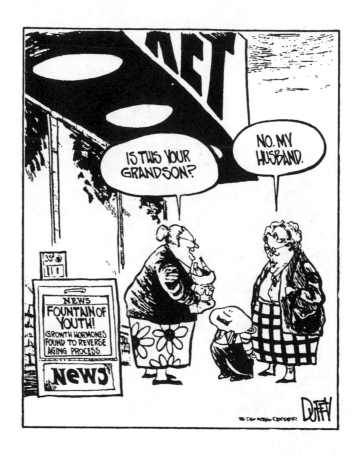

Reprinted with permission of *The Des Moines Register*.

CHAPTER ONE

Shot o' Youth, Streak o' Lean

"**W**ANTED," the ad cried out. "Healthy men between the ages of 60 and 80 years of age." Understandable. An eligible older man is hard to find. "Must live in the vicinity." Naturally; a woman can't waste precious time with the inconveniently located. "Must be available for twelve-month period." Right; weed out the ones who won't commit. "Must be no more than 20% over ideal weight." Many of the personal ads placed by men specify "slim" women only. Turn about is fair play. "Must be able to inject substance subcutaneously." Whoa. This could be a problem. "Free medical exam." OK!

An advertisement that read, well, something like that in the Chicago area newspapers, notices in the waiting rooms of area Veterans Administration (VA) Hospitals, and articles in local newspapers went on to say a medical team was looking for subjects for a study on growth hormone (GH) and its effects on aging men. No come-hither call from a middle-aged lady-in-wanting ever got such an enthusiastic response. In time a total of two hundred fifty-six bemused but eager applicants appeared on the doorstep of the North Chicago Veterans Administration Hospital. They were strapping septuagenarians in running shorts, frail men with pants hitched up over pot bellies, stocky guys who pumped iron, and bespectacled professor types. They were black, white, bald, bearded, bandannaed, embarrassed and bold. They had one thing in common: they all were interested in looking younger, feeling younger, being younger.

The medical team headed by Dan Rudman, M.D., of the Medical College of Wisconsin interviewed the 256 applicants for suitability and enrolled 95 of them for further evaluation. In the end 26 men made the cut—those whose growth hormone levels were lower than normal. For a six month base-line period, the men were tested thoroughly from head to toe, put on diets with a known distribution of protein, carbohydrate and fat and monitored to observe life-style changes. Of the twenty-one subjects who completed the baseline study, twelve subjects were randomly selected as experimental subjects to receive GH treatment by injection. Nine were designated control subjects and received no treatment. For six months, the experimental subjects gave themselves shots of GH three times a week—and waited for their muscles to pop.

The muscles didn't exactly pop. But at the end of six months, the experimental group's lean tissue—that's what the doctors call muscle—had increased 8.8%, fat tissue had decreased by 14.4%, skin had thickened up 7.1%, and back bone had become slightly stronger. "The effects of six months of growth hormone on lean body mass and adipose (fat) tissue mass were equivalent in magnitude to the changes incurred during ten or twenty years of aging," says Rudman.

Some of the experimental subjects also reported increased vigor and feelings of well-being, says Hoskote Nagraj, one of Rudman's co-investigators. "They have told their friends about their GH treatment and now their friends are coming to us asking for the treatment."

On July 5, 1990, when an article was published in the prestigious *New England Journal of Medicine* reporting the results of Rudman's study, however cautiously, the news inspired headlines all over the country: GROWTH HORMONE TURNS BACK THE CLOCK. Getting a Shot Of Youth. Injections help elderly look and feel better. More muscles, less fat. Fountain of Youth?

The flurry of headlines across the country prompted a *Des Moines Register* cartoonist to sketch a dumpy middle-aged woman telling an equally stout friend that the small baby-faced person beside her is not her grandson, but her husband. A headline on a nearby newsstand reads, "Fountain of Youth, growth hormone found to reverse aging process."

"A Good Effect All Over"

One of the rejuvenated subjects was Robert Bensing of Waukegan, Illinois. One day he saw an article in the *Waukegan News Sun* describing the proposed research of Rudman and his associates. He said he was attracted by the offer of a free medical check-up and other preventive care. All the expenses of the study were paid by research funds. The idea of maybe getting a shot of youth didn't sound half bad either, so he hustled on down to the VA Hospital in North Chicago for tests.

There he got his free physical and was found healthy. Furthermore, he was considered a desirable candidate for the study because, like almost a third of people over age 50, blood tests for a substance considered a marker for GH indicated that detectable production of GH had

11

stopped. Some of Bensing's signs of aging—decreased strength, flab around the middle, skin fragility, bone thinning—could reasonably be attributed to the cessation of GH secretion. Bensing was the almost-perfect candidate.

The only problem was he weighed more than the cut-off criterion for eligible candidates. Bensing was asked to lose 30 pounds to qualify for the program. He did and he was in.

It is appealing to imagine a fraternity of Rudman subjects, a group of stouthearted men, comparing their slimming silhouettes, new-found strength, and vitality. But this brotherhood was not meant to be. Once Bensing was in the program, he attended an orientation along with other subjects. He said hello to one or two fellows but except for a few more seminars, he did not see them again. He made appointments individually for his blood tests once or twice a month at the hospital. These were the most bothersome chores of the study. The first months were spent establishing baseline data.

The investigators considered doing a double-blind experiment in which the subjects, both experimental and control, would all take injections and neither they nor those on the research team who took measurements would know if the substance the subjects were getting was GH or a harmless, inactive solution. However, Rudman decided to pass up the experimental advantages of a double-blind study because making the control subjects go through the process of three-times-a-week injection for a year was probably too demanding. Rudman thought it would be difficult to recruit people for the project if they knew they might be in the group that went through the injections for "nothing."

The injections were no problem for Bensing. "When I was in the army getting shots, the guy next to me would faint. But I never had that problem." Though Bensing had no experience at giving injections to himself or anyone else, he says, after a couple weeks it was simple.

"You know the song about when you go to bed, you take your glass eye out, put your teeth beside the bed? Well, the shots were just one more thing like that, a chore you do for your health like brushing your teeth."

The GH came in two parts, a crystalline part and a liquid part, which had to be mixed together and injected. Both parts had to be kept refrigerated, so when he went on vacation he had to carry it in a cooler. No problem. The researchers also gave him a map of the body showing where he could stick the needle.

In fact, the difficulties of participating did not seem to daunt any of the experimental subjects. "Cooperation was fantastic," reports Dan Jackson, a VA Hospital nurse working on the study. The attrition rate was remarkable; no one dropped out of the year-long study after treatment started.

The subjects' blood levels of GH, tested indirectly, were kept within a normal range by increasing or decreasing the dose. Only four subjects required such adjustments to the original dose.

Within 24 hours after the shots began, the research team could detect signs of rebuilding lean body mass. Bensing himself began to notice "a good effect all over."

During the six-month treatment, Bensing said his muscles seemed stronger. He found he could open jars that had defied earlier attempts. He got up more easily in the morning and worked longer hours in his garden without tiring. He underwent a cataract operation, his second, and seemed to recover more rapidly than after the previous operation. Friends corroborated what he was feeling. "Boy, you look great," they said, "You seem to get younger every day." His wife, he said, could also tell the difference.

Bensing did have a bout with carpal tunnel syndrome, a painful condition of the wrist, attributed to the newly enlarged cartilage and tendons which pressed on the nerves of his wrist. The experimental subjects as a whole experienced a slight but significant rise in the average blood sugar levels and blood pressure.

Bensing and the others submitted to numerous blood tests which showed that the GH injections were working. A large caliper, whose jaws seemed more suited to measuring rhinoceros folds, recorded on a dial the increasing thickness of Bensing's once fragile skin. His bone density was evaluated, his muscles measured, his fat fathomed. Lean was up, fat was down, skin was thicker, and lower back bone was slightly denser.

Rudman relied on these objective measurements, paying relatively little attention to the subjects' own claims of strength and energy. For who could say that the knowledge of what they were taking did not make them feel stronger? Or that the attention the subjects received from the kindly staff was not what gave them their sense of well-being?

Rudman concluded that diminished secretion of growth hormone is responsible, at least in part, for the decrease of lean body mass, the expansion of fat tissue, and the thinning of skin that occur in old age. "Since atrophy of muscle and skin contributes to the frailty of older people, the potential benefits of growth hormone merit continuing attention and investigation."

He did not say, run out and get some.

When the July 5, 1990, study was published in the *New England Journal of Medicine*, reporters swarmed over the researchers. Some of the subjects were also interviewed. Bensing in particular seemed to enjoy the attention, appearing on television and in papers across the country. Project directors wanted to cool the publicity soon after Bensing mentioned to the press some data which were still being analyzed. He and other subjects were asked not to make public more details of their experience until another report of the same research could be published in *Hormone Research* near the end of 1991.

The Rudman study inspired a lot of comment from colleagues. Dr. Mary Lee Vance from the University of Virginia, in a discussion in the same issue of *The New England Journal of Medicine*, cited the Rudman study as "an important beginning in deciphering the actions of growth hormone in adults." She also mentioned the high costs of GH treatment, about $14,000 a year at present, the dangers of too much GH, and concluded, "Because there are so many unanswered questions about the use of growth hormone in the elderly and in adults with growth hormone deficiency, its general use now or in the immediate future is not justified."

And a former colleague from Rudman's Emory University days says, "Rudman is a conservative sort of fellow who wouldn't have intended to cause all this fuss in the press."

What About Me?

When news of the Rudman study broke, older people and some younger ones started pinching their fat and wondering, "What about me? I could use some of this more-muscle-less-fat stuff."

Some people called their doctors. They were told that the drug was approved by the Federal Drug Administration (FDA) but only for use in increasing the height of children with GH deficiency. Still, why not older people? I mean, if Rudman and colleagues thought it was a good idea, why wait for the plodding FDA?

Even family physicians were giving the matter serious thought. A spokesman for one of the two U.S. pharmaceutical companies that manufactures GH noticed that of the doctors calling to ask about the implications of the Rudman study, most sounded elderly. Their "I have this patient..." inquiries sounded as if the doctors were thinking of their own personal fat and lean.

In spite of the fuss this particular study caused, it was by no means the first piece of research that showed the potential of GH in shifting fat-muscle proportions though it may have been the first study on the use of GH for the elderly. Franco Salomon, M.D., and colleagues from the medical school associated with St. Thomas's Hospital in London late in 1989 had published a study on the effects of GH treatment on body composition in GH-deficient adults. The Salomon study showed that six months of treatment with GH "had a marked effect on body composition, resulting in an increase in lean body mass and a decrease in fat mass." Salomon also noted a lowered cholesterol value in the experimental subjects, an effect not found in the Rudman study.

A group of Danish investigators headed by J.O L. Jorgensen treated twenty-two GH-deficient adults, both men and women, with synthetic GH for four months. They found a significant decrease in the volume of fat on the thigh and a small increase in the strength of quadricep muscles on the front of the thigh and in capacity for exercise. These findings, reported in the summer of 1989, apparently did not find their way into headlines.

Other investigators took a look at the possibility of GH treatment of individuals who are not GH-deficient. Douglas Crist headed a research team at the University of New Mexico School of Medicine which looked at the effect of GH treatment on normal young adults who had been conditioned by years of strength training and aerobic exercise. Raising levels of GH in the blood to higher than normal levels for six weeks resulted in significantly decreased body fat and increases in fat-free weight, Crist reported in 1988.

Although such findings were published every now and then over the last few years, they did not create much of a demand for GH from ordinary people. There were individuals, however, who were quietly experiencing its effects. Thousands of unusually short children, with and without measurable GH-deficiency, were being given GH to increase their height. Many noticed other kinds of body changes. Some athletes were secretly using the substance for the same purposes as some athletes use anabolic steroids.

In the Tabloids and on the Mall

Yes, GH was known before, but the Rudman report raised public awareness of GH, and the words *growth hormone*, were popping up everywhere. "Growth Hormone makes woman grow six inches overnight," a tabloid paper screamed. A photo of a skinny woman was laid out diagonally across the front page; she grew so much she was *too long* to print straight up and down, the tabloid explained.

We discovered growth hormone while walking on the mall in front of the capitol in Washington, D.C., one sunny afternoon. We noticed a couple of young people offering drinks from a makeshift "lemonade" stand. Passers-by drank the yellow liquid from paper cups.

The literature handed out with the drink described several products including one called Be Your Best (TM). The ingredients of the Be Your Best (TM) beverage included "GH releasers," nutrients that stimulate the production of GH in the body. Human Growth Hormone, the flyer said, is "the specific hormone involved in *burning fat and building muscle.*" It went on to describe its role in resistance to disease, tissue repair, and reduction of urea in the blood. So what were the ingredients that offered us the advantages of GH in an easy-sipping drink? Vitamin-C, beta carotene, and other well-known vitamins and minerals, and—what's this?—L. arginine.

Was there something to this? Would L. arginine give *us* an extra shot of GH, a little streak 'o lean? One of us has some unwanted flab, and both of us have been known to ask ourselves, "Where's the beef?" And a few extra years of apparent youth wouldn't hurt either one of us, we thought.

We went straight to our Random House dictionary which said arginine is "one of the essential amino acids that make up plant and animal protein." Sounded OK. And then, "present in the sperm of salmon and herring."

We were halfway to the fish market before we realized that we didn't know how to tell a male salmon from a female and even if we did...well, the fish would be dead, right? We weren't sure what to do next.

So we made a quick left hand turn into The Green Green Grass of Home health food store. There we found bottle after bottle of arginine products with names like Burn 'n Build, Hot Stuff, and Mega Force "for weight lifters and athletes." Some of these supplements contained both arginine and another GH-releaser, ornithine. The latter, the Random House dictionary says, is "obtained from the hydrolysis of arginine, secreted by birds." It's nice to know that if the salmon source fails, another source is as close as our car parked under the pear tree.

With what Rudman's study showed and with GH releasers so close at hand, maybe we could be boosting our own GH without worrying about the FDA?

We confess we have been pulling your leg just a little.

We wouldn't actually try to boost our own GH levels until we got the go-ahead from a more reliable source than the headlines or a sales pitch on the mall. Neither should you. We headed over to Emory University library before jumping to conclusions or to action. We got the actual study by Rudman out of the July 5, 1990, *New England Journal of Medicine*, read it from top to bottom, even the footnotes, and digested the discussion following by Mary Lee Vance. Then we talked to some endocrinologists and read hundreds of pages of research. The endocrinologists were OK, but the research was humorless. There were ten-syllable words and initials enough to make a year's supply of alphabet soup. And yet, it was engrossing as a puzzle. We also found a historian with a sense of humor, talked to some people who grew too much and some people who grew too little, and read a lot of very cautious reports and some very serious warnings. Only then were we ready to evaluate the Fountain of Youth headlines and project what GH might mean to us—and to you.

Will growth hormone prove safe and effective long-term for GH-deficient elderly people? Can older people with normal GH levels achieve benefits similar to those of the experimental subjects? What is normal anyway? Can young adults benefit from GH? Is GH safe for them? What about short children who are not deficient in GH? Who will be allowed to take it? If it is approved for a large population, will the costs come down? Ouch! Isn't there some better way to take GH than a shot?

The answers to these questions are not currently available and even when more facts are in, professional agreement will likely not come easily. Judging the benefits and risks ourselves requires some under-standing of how hormones work, how the clinical use of hormones got to where it is today, and where GH is likely to go in the future.

Dem 'Mones, Dem 'Mones, Dem Hormones: A Very Short Course in Endocrinology

You know the spiritual that goes, "De head bone's connected to de neck bone, neck bone's connected to de shoulder bone, shoulder bone's connected to de back bone, ...Dem bones, dem bones, dem dry bones."

If the song were about hormones, singing it would be a lot more daunting. One verse might go: The sensory organs are connected to the cortex, the cortex connected to the hypothalamus, the hypothalamus connected to the pituitary, the pituitary secretes eight hormones and at least three inhibiting factors that interact with the adrenals, the thyroid, the gonads, and dozens of organs that scientists do not fully understand. Dem 'mones, dem 'mones, dem hormones.

Luckily, there is no such song. Here's what you need to know in plain prose.

21

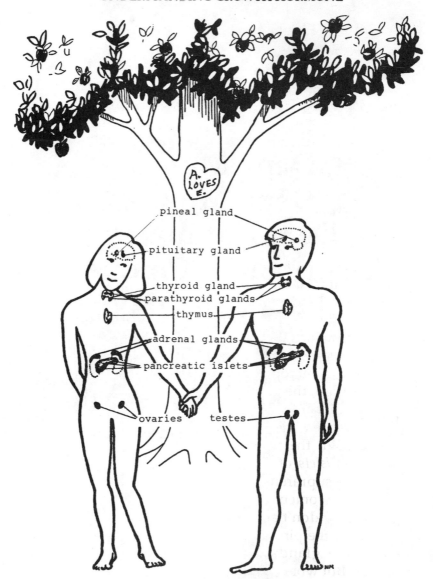

THE MAJOR ENDOCRINE GLANDS

Illustration by Nathan McKnight.

The Hormone Connection

Hormone comes from a Greek word meaning to set in motion. Hormones are biochemical substances, chemical messengers, that set in motion critical functions all over the body. Hormones are manufactured by endocrine tissue.

Endocrine refers to glands and other tissue that secrete hormones internally. Endocrine glands and other endocrine tissue, unlike *exocrine* glands, do not have special tubes or ducts to take their secretions to the next destination; endocrine tissue secretes hormones directly into the bloodstream where their influence spreads rapidly. While researchers from earliest times could easily follow exocrine substances—tears, saliva, and bile, for example, by their ducts, hormone activity was much harder to trace. Hormones, unseen in the heavy traffic of the bloodstream, were first known only by the functions they set in motion.

The *nine endocrine glands*, pictured on the facing page, are, from top to bottom: The *pineal* gland located in mid-brain, the *pituitary* (also called the hypophysis) located further forward in the brain, the *thyroid* in front of the trachea, the four *parathyroid* glands attached to the thyroid, the *thymus* right below the thyroid, the *pancreatic islets* of the pancreas, the two *adrenal* (also called the suprarenal glands) over the kidneys, the two *ovaries* in women, and the two *testes* in men. All together they don't amount to a hill of beans. The smallest gland, the pineal, is about the size of a pea; all the endocrine glands together weigh less than seven ounces. But what a wallop they pack.

The Adrenalin Rush, an Example

Adrenalin or epinephrine, from the adrenal glands is

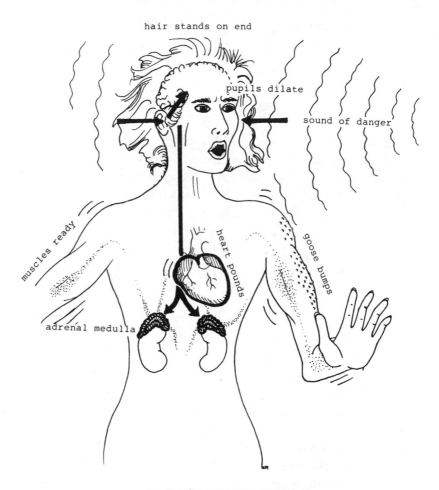

THE ADRENALIN RUSH

Sounds of danger are received by the ear then passed as nerve signals to the cortex of the brain then down the spine to the adrenal gland where the hormone adrenalin is released into the blood stream. The adrenal rush is a hormone reaction you can often feel all over your body. *Illustration by Nathan McKnight.*

a good hormone to illustrate in a vivid way how hormones work because you can sometimes actually feel it in action. Let's say your nine-year-old son says he's going out to ride his bike. You live on a cul de sac and riding the bike at your end of the street is fairly safe. Moments after the kid has slammed the front door, however, you hear the screech of brakes and a sickening thud. At that very moment, the adrenalin surges from somewhere in your gut and instantly rushes all over your body. You can feel the wave hit your arms and legs. It feels sharp and cold; your skin tingles, your heart pounds. You rush out the front door ready to pick up the car off your child's body and slam it across the road, if necessary, before you call the ambulance.

Then, on the front walk you see your son, squatting by his bike, calmly adjusting the bike chain. Both of you glare at the offending car which has just demolished your garbage can. You hug your son; you get the shakes. He wonders what's the matter with you. Back inside, you can't quite get over the scare. You are still revved up for action.

This is what happened:

A disturbance occurred outside you. Your sensory organs got a message. Your ears heard the screech and the thud and passed this information on to the cortex of your brain, the smart part that said, "Whoa...I've heard this sound before and it means big trouble." The cortex didn't dilly-dally. It sent a message down to the emergency center in the hypothalamus which sent a nerve impulse on to the adrenal medulla. The adrenalin poured into the bloodstream where it reached the heart within a fraction of a second. The heart responded instantly by speeding up and increasing its output so the message would be pushed through the bloodstream faster and harder. Increased blood pressure pushed the blood out into every little capillary till they tingled with tautness. Adrenalin also galloped by other organs. The stomach and intestines stopped their work to allow more effort in the action areas. The liver poured out extra sugar into the blood for energy in expectation of the extraordinary work that might have to be done.

You needed this pony express network to get a little action because there were many kinds of complex responses and many variations of speed to react to the outside event appropriately. Pushing one button just won't do it.

When the emergency is over, and, in this case, before the body has exhausted its resources, you still have the adrenalin in your veins, you still are pumped up. You won't be able to relax until the adrenalin has been reabsorbed by the kidney. This might be a good time to use that energy carrying old magazines down from the attic and throwing them in the trash can. Only trouble is, the trash can is mashed flat. Okay, maybe you could cut back the hedge.

Hyper, Hypo, and Hippo

When the endocrine glands are normal, everthing goes along fine. When the glands are overactive or underactive, however, strange things start to happen. An overactive or *hyper*active gland secretes too much hormone; an underactive or *hypo*active gland secretes too little. Now is a good time to get the prefixes straight.

Hyper, meaning literally too much, is often used as a slang expression to mean someone is fast-paced, excitable, super-energetic, too revved-up. Note, for example, what *Time Magazine* White House correspondent

Dan Goodgame wrote in May 1991 about President George Bush:

> The most distinctive feature of President Bush's golf game is its pace. He does everything in a hurry, from tying on his spikes to slashing the ball with his driver and chasing it at breakneck speed in his golf cart. He once played 18 holes at Cape Arundel, his home course in Kennebunkport, ME., in 1 hr. 42 min., about a third of the normal time.

The President's daily running, racquet sports, and hands-on management of the government are apparently conducted at the same frantic pace as his golf game. Bush's style could be called hyper. In fact, after an incidence of racing heart beat on May 4, 1991, the President was diagnosed as having a hyperactive thyroid and was given radioactive thyroid treatment to destroy the gland. Since then he has taken daily medication to replace the thyroid hormones at a normal level. An increase of 40% above normal in metabolic rate is considered *hyperthyroidism*. That form of hyperthyroidism, Graves' Disease, actually afflicts both President Bush and his wife Barbara. Mrs. Bush suffers from a protrusion of the eyes called *exophthalmos*, often a sign of Graves' Disease.

A decrease in thyroid hormone output to 40% below normal, on the other hand, is considered *hypothyroidism*. In a hypo state people tend to be sluggish and gain weight. Severe thyroid deficiency in adults causes *myxedema*. The disease, which afflicts more women than men, starts with slowed heart action and respiration, lowered body temperature, and lethargy and, without treatment, ends in coma, "myxedema madness," and death. A severely hypoactive thyroid during fetal life and shortly after birth results in *cretinism*, a disorder marked by mental retardation and dwarfism.

A hippo, by contrast, is a large, rotund mammal often found lolling in the shallows of African lakes.

The Pituitary: The Master Gland

The pituitary gland has been dubbed "the master gland" and "the director of the endocrine orchestra" because it produces nine known hormones, most of which stimulate the release of other hormones by other glands. The pituitary hormones that have this control over the secretions of other glands are termed *trophic hormones*. The glands influenced by the pituitary hormones are called *target glands*. But if the pituitary is the director of the orchestra, it must be acknowledged that the hypothalamus is the chairman of the board.

The *hypothalamus*, an organ in the lower part of the brain, is a control center for the autonomic nervous system and regulates the release of pituitary hormones. The hypothalamus sends several substances called *hormone releasing factors* through the pituitary stalk as messengers to the pituitary from the brain. The pituitary in response releases corresponding pituitary hormones which go on to target organs. These are often other endocrine glands with their own hormone secretions. For example, TRH (thyroid-stimulating- hormone releasing hormone) is sent from the hypothalamus to the pituitary signaling the release of TSH (thyroid stimulating hormone) from the pituitary. TSH in turn stimulates thyroid gland growth and the secretion of thyroid hormones. Indeed, growth hormone secretion is part of a similar progression of events (see the details in Chapter 4).

In addition to signaling the release of hormones, the hypothalamus sends *inhibiting factors* to the pituitary: PIF (prolactin inhibiting factor), for example, inhibits the release of prolactin, the milk-making hormone. Between stimulation and inhibition, the pituitary—the master gland—is at the beck and call of the hypothalamus.

The Feedback System

In addition to a relay system of hormone messengers, the "pony express" of the endocrine system, there is also a registered mail feature by which the receiver of the message sends back notice of receipt. For example, when the blood level of the hormone thyroxine is high enough, the thyroxine level signals to the hypothalamus to slow down, enough is enough.

The Other Lobe

Actually there are two lobes to the pituitary; all the functions mentioned above derive from the anterior or front lobe of the pituitary. The posterior or rear lobe does not produce any hormones itself but functions as a storage area and releasing agent for two hormones produced by the hypothalamus: vasopressin, an antidiuretic hormone which conserves body fluids, and oxytocin, which causes contractions of the uterus and helps in fertilization and milk production. There's the hypothalamus getting into the endocrine business again.

Pituitary disorders may start in the pituitary itself or start in the hypothalamus with much the same effects on all the glands down the chain of command. Too little pituitary activity, for example, affects the gonads (male and female sex organs) first. With too little gonadotropic stimulation, both male and female experience delayed puberty and exhibit small or atrophied sex organs. Deficiencies in other trophic hormones result in disruptions in the functioning of the target glands. The good news is that up to three-fourths of the anterior pituitary may be destroyed before major disruption of the other functions occurs. The bad news is that such destruction can be caused by radiation, surgery, syphilis, tuberculosis, hemorrhage or trauma.

The Other Endocrine Glands

The *thyroid*, a relatively large gland, secretes a number of hormones that contain the identifying element *iodine*, notably *thyroxine* and *triiodothyronine*. Body metabolism, the use of food for energy, growth, and mental development, is the major area of thyroid function.

The *parathyroid glands*, each the size of a match head, are connected to the thyroid gland. Usually they number four, but occasionally three, sometimes five or six. Parathyroid hormone (PTH) regulates levels of phosphorus, calcium, and magnesium in the blood. PTH raises the calcium level by increasing the absorption of calcium from food in the gastrointestinal tract, by decreasing the calcium excreted as waste by the kidney, and—most important—by initiating release of calcium from storage in the bone.

The *pineal gland*, perhaps the least understood of the endocrine glands, converts nerve impulses to hormonal messages. The two-lobed gland regulates functions of other endocrine glands in much the same way as the pituitary. Most of the pineal hormones, however, suppress rather than excite some function in target glands. The pineal wakes up with the sun, the strobe lights, and the burning of the midnight oil. It produces its hormones best when the light is brightest. The pineal has some heavy responsibilities nobody else would touch: it tells you when to wake up, when to go to sleep, and when to start puberty. Pineal hormones include *histamine, serotonin, melatonin* and probably many more not yet identified. Pineal secretions are of particular interest because a not-yet-isolated pineal product seems to inhibit the growth of malignant tumors.

The *thymus* is another candidate for "least understood." Its two lobes each have an inner core called the medulla and an outer covering called the cortex. This gland has a major role in developing the lymph or white blood cell system in childhood. Although thymic hormones are produced in small quantities throughout life, the thymus starts to atrophy at puberty and practically disappears in adulthood when its role is taken over by other organs. Two known hormones are *thymosin* and *thymin* which act on immune response. The thymus seems to play a part in rejecting tissue grafts and in suppressing tumors; regulation of thymic action therefore is playing an increasingly important role in the expanding technology of organ transplants and the control of cancer. The gland is also being studied as a key to autoimmune diseases like lupus, arthritis, Hodgkin's disease, and AIDS.

The *pancreatic* islands scattered within the pancreas produce the hormone *insulin*, which metabolizes sugars and fats, and the hormone *glucagon*, which also has a role in maintaining the proper levels of sugar in the blood. A disruption of insulin production results in the most common endocrine disease, *diabetes mellitus*.

The *adrenal glands* consist of two independent parts which function as separate glands. The reddish-brown *adrenal medulla*, is the source of the "adrenalin rush." Closely tied to the sympathetic nervous system, it duplicates some its functions; for that reason it is not essential for life. The adrenal medulla secretes two hormones in response to stress: *Norepinephrine* causes a rise in blood pressure and heart rate, dilates pupils, and suppresses gastro-intestinal activity. *Epinephrine*, another name for adrenalin, increases body metabolism as much as 100% and, as we have described earlier, increases amount of available sugar in muscles in preparation for increased activity, dilates heart vessels, and increases the output of the heart. The activities of both hormones favor survival in fight-or-flight situations. They get your dukes up or give wings to your heels, depending on how big the other guy is!

The *adrenal cortex*, the golden-yellow outer covering of the gland, is proportionately large in the fetus and shrinks after birth. Its function is always essential for life. It manufactures three groups of hormones called *corticosteroids*: (1) Mineralocorticoids (principally *aldosterone*) regulate sodium, potassium, and other mineral levels. (2) Glucocorticoids (principally *hydrocortisone*) control glucose levels, block inflammation, and regulate metabolism of carbohydrates, fat and protein. Glucocorticoids are well known for their use in reducing inflammation in injury or from arthritis. (3) Sex steroids (principally *androgens*) govern secondary sex characteristics. The adrenal cortex manufactures all these steroid hormones out of (Get this!) *cholesterol*. That's the nicest thing anyone has said about cholesterol since the fat hit the fan.

The *testes* of the male produce androgens, primarily *testosterone*, the hormone chiefly responsible for the development of male sex characteristics including the descent of testicles, enlargement of mature sex organs, sperm production, and sexual behavior.

The *ovaries* of the female produce the egg and secrete hormones. *Estrogen* hormones (there are at least six) stimulate growth of sex organs for reproduction and milk production. Estrogen also affects bone growth, the shape of the pelvic bone, the closing of the growth plates, fat distribution, and the condition of skin and hair. Another ovarian hormone, *progesterone*, prepares the uterus for the fertilized egg and maintains pregnancy. Estrogen and progesterone production mostly stops at menopause; hormone replacement therapy is becoming standard treatment to relieve discomforts and maintain bone strength.

The Tissue Issue

You may have noticed the term used in the beginning of this chapter, "endocrine glands and *other endocrine tissue.*" Complicating the picture of the endocrine system is the fact that some hormones are secreted into the blood stream by tissues other than the nine endocrine glands. Some mucous cells of the stomach and intestines, for example, have endocrine functions. The big three gastro-intestinal (GI) hormones are *secretin, gastrin,* and *cholecystokin-pancreozymin* (which we hope has a nickname). At least a dozen "newer" hormones of the GI tract bear long names shortened to monikers like GIP and VIP, alliterative names like pancreatic polypeptide, and others that look like names of Italian food. The placenta, the protective, nurturing organ surrounding a fetus, also acts as endocrine tissue, producing the hormone progesterone and other substances necessary for the development of the fetus. Even the fat of an obese woman can be a minor source of estrogen after ovaries have stopped producing the female hormone at menopause. The heart and the lungs also have been found to secrete hormones, and the versatile hormones called *prostaglandins* are almost everywhere, secreted by many different kinds of cells.

Another source of confusion is that an endocrine gland can have additional exocrine functions. The testes, for example, secrete and release the hormone testosterone—without ducts—a purely endocrine function; at the same time, the glands' other products, semen and sperm, are released through a duct—an exocrine activity.

How Do We Know All This?

Such a tangle of relationships among substances and organs was a real bear for medical researchers. Nothing like the knee bone connected to the shin bone. The study of hormones known as endocrinology began in prehistory, gathered momentum during the Renaissance, and exploded in complexity in the twentieth century when hundreds of hormones have been discovered. Between prehistory and the twentieth century a fascinating story was unfolding, one of observation and experiment, trial and error, argument and agreement, all leading in the direction of successful treatment.

CHAPTER THREE

Hurried Hormone History

The development of growth hormone therapy is almost entirely a twentieth-century accomplishment but one grounded in the investigations of the distant past. Doctors, philosophers, and professors of anatomy as well as an occasional sculptor, draper, or lens grinder had prodded, poked, powdered, and sliced the organs of man and other animals since the beginning of history. They had measured and maneuvered, tested and tasted, dyed and traced the strange substances that flowed out of certain organs called

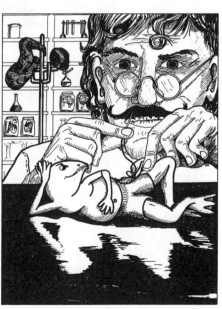

Illustration by Nathan McKnight.

glands until, by the twentieth century, they knew pretty much what they were looking for. The modern saga of growth hormone depends on the ancient history of endocrinology. To skim the top of this rich body of knowledge, we used Victor Medvei's fascinating and exhaustive *A History of Endocrinology* as our major source.

The Archeology of Endocrinology

People in ancient civilizations had observed the function of the endocrine system and, perhaps more important, the disfunction of the endocrine system since the beginning of humankind. Painters, sculptors, potters and scribes were not only artists but record keepers serving as amazingly accurate medical illustrators of the distortions of disease.

Diseases of endocrine origin were described or depicted by ancient civilizations all over the world. Portraits of Tutankhamen, famed fourteenth-century Egyptian king (or was it a queen?), illustrate features and proportions that may have indicated *intersex*, a sexual ambiguity caused by disruptions of sex hormones. A first-century B.C. carving of the otherwise beautiful Queen Cleopatra shows an enlarged area on the neck that may have been goiter. A limestone portrait of King Akhenaten (Amenhotep IV) dating from 1365 B.C. suggests the structures of the royal face were distorted by too much growth hormone. Dwarfs stunted by a variety of disorders enlivened Egyptian tomb paintings.

Ayur Veda, the art of Hindu medicine from the period between 1400 and 400 B.C., describes a disease known as "honey urine," which we now understand to be diabetes mellitus, a disturbance in insulin production which causes sugary wastes to pass in the urine. A prehistoric Peruvian jug formed in the shape of a person's head features severely bulging eyes, a symptom of Graves disease.

Hare's Brain, Wolf's Liver

Ancient treatment of endocrine diseases, though hardly universally effective, foreshadowed modern hormone replacement. Ancients performed organ magic or, to give it a more pretentious name, organotherapy: They frequently prescribed eating an organ of an animal—or in the case of cannibals, of a friend or an enemy—to replace the functioning of an ailing organ. Pliny the Elder, for one, a Roman scholar who died in the 79 A.D. eruption of Mount Vesuvius, recommended animal organ therapy, like for like: testicles of animals to cure male sexual dysfunction, genitalia of female animals to get pregnant, hare's brains for nervous disorders, wolf's liver for hepatitis, spleen for ailing spleen. A medieval Chinese account from 1475 A.D. reports this treatment: take the thyroid glands of pigs, dry them, then powder them, and administer with wine. This method of "taking thyroid" apparently worked to some degree. Such treatments supplied nutrients in which the patient could have been deficient and may have provided actual hormone replacement.

Seventeenth-century London drug catalogs called pharmacopoeia offered an impressive list of products for organotherapy—bile, blood, bones, brains, claws, eggs, excrement, eyes, feathers, placenta, and urine from a variety of animals. It sounds like the same catalogue where Macbeth's witches shopped for their "eye of newt and toe of frog, wool of bat and tongue of dog." Indeed, medicine and magic were thinly divided in Shakespeare's time.

Urine therapy in China between the eleventh and the

seventeenth centuries went one step further. Therapeutic quantities of products were extracted from huge amounts of human urine. (Picture the process of collecting 200 gallons of urine at one time!) The urine was crystallized or dried to powder form; also proteins could be precipitated out of the urine using available chemicals. The recovered proteins probably included the sex-related hormones androgen and estrogen, the adrenal hormones norepinephrine and adrenalin, and other bio-chemical substances. Treatment with these products suggested, if not true understanding of hormones, at least a complex, empirical foray into hormone replacement.

And did the early Chinese know that thyroid goiter was often caused by a lack of iodine in the diet? Or was a cure discovered by chance when a shore-dwelling Chinaman happened to lug a bucket of iodine-rich seaweed from the ocean to his mountain cousin who suffered from goiter? In any case, an account dated 340 A.D. indicates the Chinese, long before Europeans, used seaweed to treat the disease, common in those mountain areas where sources of iodine were scarce.

Keen observation probably prompted most practices of ancient hormonal manipulation. Egyptian mothers, for instance, were directed by experts to breastfeed their babies for over two years to reduce fertility and space children the preferred three years apart. The experts did not necessarily know that prolactin, the milk-making hormone, worked to inhibit ovulation. Ancient Egyptians also surgically removed the ovaries of human females as a means of contraception without knowing how the ovaries made pregnancy possible.

Medicine in Temple and Toga:
Greek and Roman Thinking

Over the centuries, isolated observations and empirical cures were drawn together by scholars and physicians to form the science, philosophy, or art of medicine. The ancient Chinese, Egyptians, and Hindus all made noteworthy contributions to medical thought. The Greeks, however, provided the most influential antecedents to modern Western medicine. The Greeks had a long medical tradition which began with certain gods as healers. Temples to these gods were tended by priest-physicians and became seats of physicians' guilds and health centers. It is the sacred snakes of these temple cults that appear coiled around the staff of the caduceus, emblem of the medical profession.

Hippocrates (460-370 B.C.), known as the father of Western medicine, was born into a family of temple physicians. Hippocrates applied logic, independent of religion and philosophy, to long years of detailed clinical observation. His notes included descriptions of many endocrine diseases and the circumstances under which they occur.

Medicine was practiced in Greece not only by temple physicians but by gymnasts, scholars, philosophers, and do-it-yourselfers. One philosopher-mathematician-physician, Pythagoras (580-489 B.C.), best known for his theorem concerning right triangles, had several ideas that foreshadowed hormones under the control of the hypothalamus. He was the first to regard the brain as the main organ of higher activities. He also brought from Egypt and further developed the idea of *humors*. Besides the four major humors observable in the body—blood, phlegm, yellow bile, and black bile— other humors were thought to travel through the nervous system which ancient people had already traced. Many changes in emotional state, health, and behavior were ascribed to the ebb and flow of these substances. An expression such as "in a bad humor," is a remnant of the theory of humors which was prevalent for two thousand years from about 500 B.C. through the end of the eighteenth century. Besides the four humors, Pythagoras considered the four qualities—dry, moist, hot, cold—which added to the four elements—earth, air, fire, and water—gave a set of twelve which could be combined in endless proportions and whose balance or imbalance could explain health and disease.

Famed Greek philosopher Aristotle (384-322 B.C.) complicated medical arts with another set of four—the four causes—matter, mover, form, and end. He regarded the brain as a gland secreting cold humors to balance hot humors from the heart. (Cool head over warm heart?) An astute naturalist, Aristotle studied the daily development of chick embryos and wrote the first Greek description of contraception. When observing that obese women often could not conceive and very skinny ones had no menses, he was unknowingly describing endocrine disorders.

Greek observations were extensive and not without error. Pre-Aristotle theorists thought genetic material came from the father only. Others believed that the right testicle produces male sperm and the left testicle female and that tying off one testicle would determine the sex of baby. Apparently no one was game to test this theory experimentally.

In fact, the Greeks of the Golden Age were long on observation and thought and short on lab time to prove a theory experimentally.

In the period between 156-576 A.D., when the Greeks and Romans pooled their talents, knowledge of the endocrine system became more precise. The ideas of Galen (130-200 A.D.), a transplanted Greek who practiced in Rome, seem particularly modern. In *De Voce* he wrote of the double-lobed thyroid, "The neck has two glands" with "no ducts through which the humors may flow, as is the case in the two glands of the tongue. But those which are in the neck are of a spongy nature and from those the humor oozes out and trickles down, there being no necessity for ducts (which the others need) whereby the fluid may be carried." In describing this absence of ducts, Galen thus noted the defining characteristic of the endocrine system. Galen also knew of the pituitary and thymus glands.

Knife, Lens, Ink, and Taffeta Tights: The Renaissance and Age of Reason

When the Middle Ages set in, preservation of past knowledge was the main order of scholarship. Galen and Aristotle remained for centuries the most respected authorities on medicine until the Renaissance brought a spirit of inquiry and increasing practice of an old technique for anatomical learning, the *post mortem* dissection of the human body. Famed Roman artist cum scientist Leonardo da Vinci (1452-1519) made his anatomical drawings at the dissection table. Andreas Vesalius (1514-1564) was also a first rate dissector. His descriptions of the thyroid gland, the ovaries, and the pituitary were landmark works. He gave the pituitary its name but missed its function, concluding that this important gland secreted mucus to the nose. Renaissance scientists were very big on tracing tubes for fluids; Fallopius and Eustachi both got tubes named for them.

The search for clues to the endocrine system was given another big boost with the invention of the microscope by Galileo in 1609. Robert Hooke made the first really workable lenses in mid-century and was the first to describe cells in the tissue of living things. Then everyone got into the act. A draper cum scientist from Delft named Leeuwenhock (1632-1723) had a passion for lenses which he ground himself. Through his lens one day Leeuwenhock's student discovered sperm, "little animals" which Leeuwenhock studied at their peak of activity "within six heartbeats of ejaculation." It might seem those time constraints placed a strain on the scientist, but rabbits were marvelously obliging. Leeuwenhock went on to trace the course of the sperms' journey up the reproductive system by cutting open the hapless rabbits at different intervals after copulation and locating active sperm.

It had for a long time been thought that humors traveled via the nervous system. When it was discovered that nerves were not tubes and could not carry fluids, the whole idea of humors was questioned—but not replaced. The travels of the elusive humors were mostly matters of speculation until someone thought to trace their passageways by injecting ink or colored fluids into organs being studied. Injection was especially important to famed seventeenth-century physician William Harvey (1578-1657), the first to accurately describe and map in detail the circulatory system. The new understanding of the vast blood circulation offered the possibility of a distribution system for humors or their successors through the blood. By the middle of the seventeenth century scientists generally made a distinction between exocrine and endocrine glands according to whether their secretions were delivered to specific location by ducts or released directly into the blood.

Throughout the eighteenth century the poking and

prodding, slicing and dyeing continued unabated. The connection between the thymus and the lymph system was discovered—and argued. The thyroid remained a mystery although one leader in endocrinology opined, "that the use of the gland is very considerable may appear from the largeness of the arteries which it receives from the carotid." A connection was discovered between the pituitary and the hypothalamus through the pituitary stalk. The stages of ovulation were distinguished.

Diseased glands were examined for their relationship to symptoms. A pituitary tumor was linked with abnormal cessation of menstruation. High blood sugar with diabetes was linked to injury of the pancreas. The frequency of cretinism in certain mountainous regions was investigated and explained erroneously as the result of drinking melted snow or breathing stagnant valley air. A German surgeon, Lorenz Heisler (1683-1758), observed that people often considered the abnormal but common growth, goiter, on the neck an ornament. Either for that reason, poverty, or fear of surgery, people often left them unattended until they sometimes reached "such a degree that they can extend to the navel even down to the knee." By mid-eighteenth century Heisler was removing them surgically whenever he got the chance.

Some investigators went to extraordinary lengths to discover how an endocrine system worked. An Italian scientist, Lazzaro Spallanzani (1729-1799), studying the fertilization of frog eggs, made tiny tight-fitting taffeta pants to put on male frogs before copulation. The eggs released by the female did not develop, wherefore Spallanzani concluded the male frog's sperm were a necessary ingredient for reproduction. Spallanzani went on to do the first artificial insemination on a dog and on an insect. On an insect? Yes, a man who could make size 1/100 taffeta tights for a frog could probably do artificial insemination on an insect.

It might seem early scholars were disproportionately interested in sexual functions. But note that the reproductive system was one that went through dramatic observable cycles in a fairly short length of time; the male organs were easy to get at, and the reproductive system also was the only one that could be altered experimentally without killing or ruining the health of a human subject. Medvei goes so far as to title one chapter of his *A History of Endocrinology*, "The Oldest Key to the Endocrine Treasure Trove: The Testicles."

In spite of the extensive knowledge of testicles the ancients had, it took until the nineteenth century for an experiment in the modern sense to be performed.

It is one thing to observe and draw conclusions. It is another to manipulate variables, holding others constant, and then to observe and draw conclusions. This is one great contribution of the nineteenth century: the experimental method.

Professor Berthold's Roosters Announce the Dawn of Experimental Medicine

Professor Arnold Berthold kept a few chickens at his home in Gottingen, Germany. No doubt the neighbors were wakened by crowing early in the morning, but there in the privacy of his backyard at least the professor could easily perform experiments unnoticed. Frankly, he was afraid his colleagues at the university would ridicule him if they knew what he was doing with his cackling Leghorns.

Like the ancients, Berthold knew that castrating or removing the gonads of a rooster changed the animal dramatically. Castrated roosters were called capons.

The caponized birds became fat and lazy afterwards and did not act like roosters. Berthold wanted to know why.

In 1848 he removed the sex glands from four young roosters. He put two of the birds back out in the barnyard. They were the control subjects. He did something extraordinary to the other two, the experimental subjects. He cut open their abdomens, grafted a single testicle inside, and sewed them up. The experimental subjects were soon out in the barnyard with the others where Professor Berthold pulled up a chair and began some serious bird watching.

What he noticed was that the caponized control roosters soon grew fat and lazy, just right for eating. Their bright red combs faded and shrank. They stopped crowing and stopped chasing hens. In short, they behaved like capons have always behaved.

The experimental roosters, however, with the transplanted testicle stuffed inside, never got the message that they were no longer roosters. They pranced and crowed, chased hens, fought off rival roosters. Their combs stood up stiff and bright. They behaved like roosters have always behaved.

In due time, Professor Berthold decided to look into the situation. He killed the two strutting roosters and looked inside to see what the transplanted sex organs were doing. He found that the testicles had sprouted a few capillaries and connected themselves to the roosters' circulatory systems. He did not find that any nerve regeneration had occurred. This was an important point because up until then scientists had thought that behavior was controlled by the nervous system. Berthold demonstrated that some substance generated in the gonads operated, not through nerves, but via the blood stream, and that this substance was directly responsible for male secondary sex characteristics.

Actually Berthold was not the first to transplant testicles. The versatile genius John Hunter (1728-1793) had performed a similar transplantation of a cock's testes to the abdomen of a hen as early as 1771, but Hunter, at that point, was more interested in studying grafting than in drawing conclusions about how gonads influence secondary sexual characteristics. Berthold, by contrast, manipulated variables, used control subjects, and interpreted the results of his experiment in a landmark conclusion.

Berthold went public with his findings in a treatise published in the *Archives of Anatomy, Physiology, and Medical Science,* but the news caused no great change in scientific thinking at the time, perhaps because a few other researchers were unable to successfully repeat the experiment. Indeed, it is remarkable that any such transplantation had succeeded, conducted as it was in ignorance of bacterial inflammation, atrophy from oxygen deficiency, and tissue rejection by the immune system. Berthold's classic experiment is now considered the first sound experimental knowledge of the circulation of hormones through the bloodstream to set in motion activity throughout the body, i.e., the role which defines hormones.

Berthold, apparently taken with birds, went on to write a thesis on thyroids of green parrots. Other nineteenth-century bird watchers, describing birds with male plumage on one side and female plumage on the other, connected this rare condition with corresponding one-sided abnormalities of the sex organs. The intensified search for such connections between disorder and a diseased gland was, along with the experimental method, a critical step towards usable endocrinology in the nineteenth century.

Doctor Thomas Addison and the Shriveled Gland

The same year that Berthold did the testicle switch, Dr. Thomas Addison, a "proud and pompous" physician at Guy's Hospital in London, made a discovery that immeasurably advanced the study of endocrinology. Addison was known for his phenomenal attention for detail and his unfailing memory. He collected data in his head about subtle symptoms of his patients. He began to notice a syndrome of symptoms in patients dying a familiar lingering death.

In autopsies he discovered that the glands on top of the kidneys, which he called the supra-renal capsules, were atrophied; in one case that was the only lesion in the body. Addison, "a careful and patient man," treated and autopsied eleven other patients with the same set of symptoms over a period of five years before he declared publicly that he had discovered a previously unknown disease directly associated with the atrophy of the supra-renal capsules, now known as the supra-renal glands or, more commonly, the adrenal glands. He achieved a certain fame when the disease, an insufficiency of adrenal functioning, was permanently dubbed Addison's disease.

The White House Disease

Robert James Graves (1796-1853) accurately described in detail a disease presenting protruding eyes and heart palpitations and correctly attributed these symptoms to an enlarged thyroid gland. It was duly named Graves Disease in 1860 for the astute researcher. Graves Disease has become a household word since

President Bush and his wife were diagnosed, but the same syndrome also goes by at least twenty other names.

Pigs Adrenals, Dog Testes: A Reprise

A third contribution of nineteenth-century endocrinology was not new but renewed interest in an ancient practice, organotherapy, with a new wrinkle—injection.

The peripatetic physician Charles Brown-Sequard (1817-1894), after high-profile careers in France, United States, England, and France again, proposed that the testes contained an invigorating substance which could be injected into men to rejuvenate them and aid in the treatment of all manner of illnesses. At the age of 72, the good doctor tried out on himself a few injections of dog testicle, crushed whole then filtered. A delighted Brown-Sequard noted, "the very considerable changes which have been produced in my body," which he denied were autosuggestion after achieving a similar rejuvenation of a number of patients. Organotherapy became the rage. *The British Medical Journal* was concerned, Medvei tells us, complaining that "The statements [Brown-Sequard] made—which have unfortunately attracted a good deal of attention in the public press—recall the wild imaginings of medieval philosophers in search of an elixir vitae."

The same—in so many words—has been said about popular coverage of the Rudman growth hormone study.

Wild imaginings or not, the idea of organotherapy was much in the forefront. In 1891 Brown-Sequard and a colleague had, as Medvei reports, "argued that potent substances must exist in animal tissues, the process (and the result) of 'internal secretion.' These substances

48

could be discovered by using extracts obtained from specific tissue for the treatment of certain diseases which are perhaps due to deficiency of an internal secretion."

The same year George Murray (1865-1939) proposed replacement therapy for myxedema using an extract from sheep's thyroid. Over the objections of colleagues, he began treatment of a 46-year-old woman. She improved dramatically and went on to receive injections until her death at age 74. Fortunately Murray had made prior arrangements with a slaughterhouse, because the lady ended up taking the equivalent of 870 sheep's thyroids. Murray's treatment became, Medvei says, "the first generally recognized success of organotherapy" and the antecedent of all the life-saving and life-enhancing hormone replacement treatment since, including insulin treatment of diabetics, estrogen replacement therapy, and yes, treatment with growth hormone.

Oliver Interrupts an Experiment

About the same time, George Oliver (1841-1915) had been experimenting with extracts of several glands, dissolved in glycerin and administered by mouth. He had invented also a device to accurately measure blood pressure and an arteriometer to measure the diameter of arteries. He had discovered that the administration of material from the adrenal glands had an effect on blood pressure and on the size of the vessels and the tone of the circulatory system. In 1893 Oliver went up to London to consult Edward Schaefer, professor of physiology at University College. Schaefer had heard about this organ extract business and was not much interested in them in general, and that day in particular, because he was very busy doing an experiment on a dog and regretted the interruption. As part of the experiment Schaefer was making repeated measures of the dog's blood pressure. Oliver, ever tactful, indicated he had no intention of interrupting such important work. But, he inquired, when Schaefer had completely finished the experiments, might he consider trying on the dog an adrenal extract which Oliver just happened to carry in his pocket?

What happened next comes from Sir Henry Dale's account of the occasion quoted in Medvei: "And so, just to convince Oliver that it was all nonsense, Schaefer gave the injection, and then stood amazed to see the mercury mounting in the arterial manometer until the recording float was lifted almost out of the distal limb." This was the first discovery of a specific physiological response to an endocrine extract.

When Schaefer had been convinced that adrenal extracts sent blood pressure out of sight, he agreed to collaborate with Oliver and the two went on to many discoveries in the field of endocrinology. Two American doctors, John Jacob Abel (1857-1938) and Albert Crawford, in 1897 at Johns Hopkins University obtained the active principle of the adrenal gland, which Abel called epinephrine (adrenalin). This was the first isolation of an endocrine secretion as a chemically pure substance and the only hormone isolated before the twentieth century.

Spirited Arguments and Colorful Discoveries

The nineteenth century, all in all, might be summed up as a hundred years of spirited debate and colorful discoveries: Purple fumes rising over seaweed ashes led to the discovery in 1811 of a new element, iodine, vital to thyroid function. An emerald green hue appeared when perchloride of iron was applied to the adrenal medulla and became a test for a substance (adrenalin) exclusively associated with the adrenals. In 1827 Carl von Baer (1792-1876) discovered the mammalian ovum, and in 1843 Martin Barry for the first time caught a sperm and egg in the act. In 1896 the existence of ovarian hormones was proven. The discovery of chromosomes opened up a new field: genetics. In 1886 Joseph von Mering (1849-1908) and Oscar Minkowski (1858-1931) produced diabetes in a dog experimentally by removing the pancreas. Two years later Minkowski caused experimental diabetes in another dog by removing its pancreas—and then cured the dog by re-implanting the excised organ. And near the end of the century, two new endocrine glands, the last of the big nine, were discovered—the pancreatic islands and the parathyroids.

The twentieth century dawned with its work cut out for it. American Nobel prize winner Edward Doisy, born in Illinois in 1893, outlined four stages of advances in endocrinology as follows (from Medvei):

1) Recognition of the gland or organ as one producing internal secretion.
2) Methods of detecting internal secretion
3) Preparation of extracts leading to a purified hormone.
4) The isolation of the pure hormone, determination of its structure and its synthesis.

The nineteenth century had much success with the first step, some small success with the second. It was left to the twentieth century to complete the tasks that would make all that went before clinically useful.

CHAPTER FOUR

Growth Hormone

Growth hormone, isolated in animals in 1945 and in humans in 1956, was originally thought to be of value only during the growing years when it causes skeletal growth. A medical book published as recently as 1972 states, "Growth hormone is not essential to health in adult life."

But Hollywood knew better. In the 1960s men, women, and children broke the humdrum of daily life by stretching out in front of the television set and watching the flickering black and white of a horror movie rerun. One ghoulish production featured a gang of murderers who killed their victims for the tiny amounts of growth hormone to be harvested from their pituitary glands. The GH was used to restore the elderly gang leader to youthfulness, an imagined purpose which foreshadowed the promise of the 1990 Rudman study.

It is now known, even outside Hollywood, that GH plays an important role in the maintenance of organs throughout life. GH is not only responsible for skeletal growth, but the growth and constant repair of many organs from the bones to the kidneys and of many systems affecting everything from metabolism to immune response.

GH, The Inside Story

GH, like other hormones, is a water soluble neurotransmitter, a biological communicator, that travels through the bloodstream to every part of the body. GH is a single chain polypeptide or complex protein, that is, (for those of you who like to make biological cell models out of marshmallows and toothpicks) its molecule is one long string of 191 amino acids (these are your marshmallows), with two bi-sulphide bonds (extra toothpicks) between molecules. Circulating GH is associated with a binding protein, a substance that will help it hook up with a specific receptor of a target organ cell.

GH is not just one substance but several related forms whose differences are observed in their molecular weight. The most important form, for example, has a molecular weight of 22,000 while its principal pituitary variant has a molecular weight of 20,000. Differences in weight may be associated with slightly different functions, for example, one variation of hGH produced by the human placenta, the organ that surrounds and nurtures the unborn child in the womb, may have a special role during pregnancy.

Scientists have studied the GH of man, monkey, ox, sheep, horse, pig, dog, rat, rabbit, and—for a special challenge—whale. The average molecular weight of these animals' GH was 22,000, the same as the main form of human GH.

Rhesus monkey GH is, in fact, active in humans and vice versa. Human GH is also active in other mammals but the reverse is not true. If such small differences in GH structure distinguish the species, variations of the same degree may well distinguish different roles through different receptors in the human body.

A Peculiar and Inaccessible Structure

All these esoteric details were fodder for researchers of the last quarter century, whose acquaintance we have made chiefly through Medvei's *A History of Endocrinology.*

In the nineteenth century and even into the twentieth, GH was unknown and the pituitary, the GH factory, was just "a peculiar and inaccessible structure," as one surgeon put it, nestled in a bony nook called the *sella turcica.* The sella turcica, early researchers had found, was like a tiny saucepan, holding the pituitary safe above the void of the nasal sinus. Measuring, in the male, about 1.5 centimeters by 1.0 centimeter, the pituitary looked like a tiny bean beginning to sprout, a big brown comma, or a newly hatched tadpole chasing its tail.

The word *pituitary* came from the Latin word *pituita,* which meant phlegm, one of the humors (the stuff in the back of your nose that you spit when you have a cold). For 1500 years it was thought that the pituitary was the source of the icky drip. "You mean, pituitary comes from *p-tui!*" one of our friends exclaimed, making the comic strip version of the spitting sound. Although we can't confirm this derivation, we find it compelling.

Apart from creating a need for spitting, the pituitary was, before the twentieth century, considered "as a mere vestigial relic of prehistoric usefulness." In 1889 an anatomist informed a group of his peers that the pituitary "has little, or perhaps no, use in the organism of higher vertebrates."

A few oddities, to be sure, had been observed about

the pituitary—its increased size during pregnancy had been noted, and an enlargement of the gland was reported among members of a Russian religious sect who had ritually castrated themselves. Tumors had been found on the pituitary, but these were not understood to relate to any particular condition. In 1892 it was demonstrated that destruction of the pituitary caused a disturbance in water and mineral metabolism. Still the basic question remained: What did the pituitary do?

The most expedient way to determine the gland's use seemed to be to remove the gland from an experimental animal and see what happened. This was attempted numerous times in the 1880s. Because of the complexity of the blood supply to the gland and its awkward position in the lower brain, what usually happened was the experimental animal died during the operation from brain damage or loss of blood.

Harvey Cushing (1869-1939), famed neurosurgeon at Johns Hopkins University and later Harvard, operated experimentally on 100 dogs using a more accurate surgical technique he had developed. Some of the dogs survived and some died, but Cushing noted that removal of the posterior pituitary did not cause death if the anterior was intact. Although some researchers had distinguished two lobes of the pituitary by the difference in their looks, Cushing's observation was the first functional distinction between the anterior and posterior lobes.

In 1908, however, the renowned but skeptical Edward Schaefer once again described the anterior pituitary as not having any physiological effect at all.

The anterior pituitary was a special interest of Bernhard Aschner (1883-1960). A Viennese surgeon who later moved to the United States when Hitler took over his country, Aschner pioneered an approach to the pituitary from the mouth through the sphenoid bone for unprecedented surgical precision. Using this technique, Aschner did 120 careful experiments with dogs and puppies between 1908 and 1912 by which he demonstrated that the anterior pituitary had a critical role in growth.

The same year before an assembly of the American Medical Association, Cushing introduced the terms *hypo-* and *hyper-* pituitarism meaning underactive and overactive pituitary function.

The Big Band Era

Over the next twenty years a big change was taking place in medical research that would boost the rate of discovery and breadth of understanding. Instead of lone researchers watching their chickens or poring over their microscopes, large research teams were pulled together in lavishly equipped research centers where neuroscientists, geneticists, biophysicists and the like could all work together in broad areas and readily share their knowledge. At the forefront of this movement was Herbert Evans.

When Evans, early in his career, turned from clinical medicine to medical research, his disappointed father, a surgeon, referred to him derisively as "my son, the rat doctor." Evans soon became famous for what he learned from rats.

In 1915 Evans was called from Johns Hopkins University to head up the then undistinguished anatomy department at his alma mater, University of California. There at Berkeley, Evans was one of the first to pull together a super-team of gifted men and women who among them could cover the wide range of knowledge that is now inextricably tied to endocrinology. Out of this group evolved the Institute of Experimental Biology.

Evans was the first to postulate a specific growth-stimulating substance released by the anterior pituitary. In 1921 Evans prepared an extract of crushed anterior pituitary tissue from cows and injected the "opaque pink fluid" into rats. Within three months "an outspoken acceleration of growth" demonstrated the presence of what we now call GH. Going one step further, another team member, biologist Philip Smith (1884-1970) excised the anterior pituitary of rats so carefully that they were devoid of all anterior pituitary hormone function, then he gave fresh extracts from the gland to the rats. The treatments not only kept the rats alive but restored growth and even produced *gigantism*. Also, Smith noted, the anterior pituitary treatment *reduced flabbiness*.

In 1929 the existence of a group of lactogens or milk-producing hormones, also secreted by the pituitary gland, was recognized. This discovery became a source of confusion in that GH is very similar in structure to the lactogenic hormones like prolactin and *choriosomatomammatropin* (at ten syllables, a new record). The various forms of GH are so similar in structure to the lactogenic hormones that it was hard to distinguish activities of the two in bioassays. In fact, the two hormone groups were treated as one until in 1933 Oscar Riddle, a bird physiologist from Indiana, identified prolactin after studying pigeon's milk (but that's a different story). In most mammals including man, lactogenic hormones are weak growth promoters and GH is a weak milk-promoter. The two hormone groups apparently have evolved from common ancestral molecules.

C.H. Li: The Patriarch of GH

One of Evans's team was Choh Hao Li. Born in 1913 into a large family of scholars in Canton, China, Li, a graduate of the University of Nanking, came to the University of California in 1935. Three years later, with a Ph.D. in physico-organic chemistry, Li sought work in Evans' Institute of Experimental Biology. In a tiny basement laboratory dominated by plumbing, Evans put Li to work painstakingly isolating the anterior pituitary hormones from animal extracts. Li chalked up the isolation of luteinizing hormone (LH) in 1940 and adrenocorticotrophic hormone (ACTH) in 1943. In 1945 Li isolated GH in amorphous form. (A crystalline form was isolated in 1949 by Wilhelmi and colleagues.) Follicle stimulating hormone (FSH) followed in 1949. Then Li put these hormones, one by one and in various combinations, back into the rats whose anterior pituitary had been excised, characterizing more fully the biological purpose of each.

In the course of such brilliant success, Li had been invited up from the basement to join the faculty. In 1950 the Board of Regents made him director of the new Hormone Research Laboratory at Berkeley, which in 1967 was moved to University of California in San Francisco.

Intense, single-minded, and competitive as a researcher, Li, known as C.H. by his colleagues, was also personable and kind as a mentor. Somewhat shy in groups perhaps because of his heavy Chinese accent, he is remembered by his students and co-workers as dynamic in the laboratory. Although he preferred to be engrossed in cells and molecules, he was also talented at managing the lab and getting it funded.

In 1955, C.H. Li isolated and purified human GH

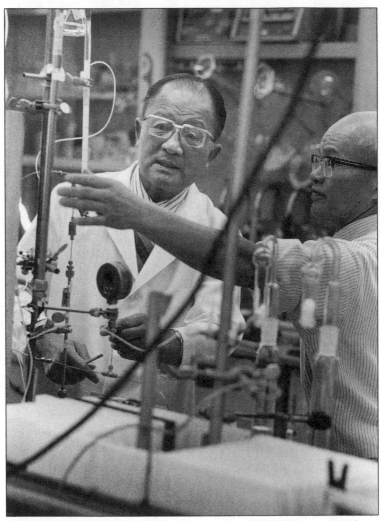

Dr. Choh Hao Li (left), 1913-1987, a biochemist at University of California, San Francisco, was credited with synthesizing most of the pituitary hormones including growth hormone. *UCSF photo by David Powers, 1979; used with permission.*

(written hGH when necessary to differentiate it from GH from other sources) from the pituitary glands of human cadavers. This was the breakthrough that made GH-replacement therapy possible.

For the next two decades Li worked on discovering the biochemical molecular structure of the anterior pituitary hormones. He had a leading role in the isolation and purification of eight of the nine anterior pituitary hormones now known.

Having discovered the structure of hGH, Li, along with chemist Donald Yamashiro, started chemically building the GH molecule from scratch, putting together amino acids, the building blocks of proteins, into groups called peptides. The first ones were only fragments of the GH molecule. Next he put these fragments into longer and longer peptide chains until, in 1971, when the 191th amino acid fell into place, it was champagne time. The GH molecule, the largest protein molecule to be synthesized up to that time, was complete.

While Li was putting the synthetic GH chain together, others were making headway with the natural stuff. Professors Knobil and Greep showed that GH extracts from monkeys were active in man while extracts from non-primates were not. In 1957 Maurice S. Raben of Tufts University Medical School used pituitary-derived hGH to make an abnormally short, GH-deficient boy grow six times as fast as he had been growing. By the mid-1970s hGH had been collected from 82,500 human pituitary glands and was being used to treat about 3000 very short children with proven GH deficiency.

Too Little, Too Late

In some ways the question of GH deficiency was

moot because whether there was deficiency or not, there was not enough pituitary GH to go around to all the GH deficient children. Only a tiny amount could be gleaned from each human pituitary, and donated tissues became increasingly hard to come by. As a result, treatment was not extended to all those who might have benefitted. Only children with no detectable GH production were given treatment. No partial deficiency was acknowledged. It was this lack of GH for treatment that originally defined GH deficiency. Moreover, those GH-deficient children who received treatment were generally denied it once they reached a "normal" height of five feet.

The DNA Revolution

With the discovery and structural characterization of DNA, linear chains of substances that make up genes, the field of genetics exploded. Genetic engineering developments in the 1970s revolutionized medical science. Identifying the components and building a complex protein as Li did, a tedious decade-long process of chemical synthesis, could now be bypassed. Through genetics the protein could be reproduced biologically. When the gene that encoded a given protein had been identified and isolated, a recombinant DNA molecule containing that gene could be constructed and then inserted into a host microorganism. The host, often the humble bacteria, escherichia coli (e. coli), then propagated or cloned the desired protein. Biosynthetic hGH could now be made in unlimited quantities.

Between the development of this possibility and the approval of the biosynthetic product for use by the Federal Food and Drug Administration (FDA), many children were getting too old to benefit from the new technology.

Then in the spring of 1985 two cases of Creutzfeldt-Jakob disease, caused by a rare and slow-acting but deadly virus in the brain, were discovered among individuals who had been treated with pituitary GH in the 1960s and 1970s. More cases were to follow. The discovery of viral contamination of the donor tissue struck a fatal blow to pituitary GH therapy. Even though improved preparation methods had made GH products purer after 1971, the FDA immediately banned all use of GH from cadavers as more cases surfaced. Fortunately, in October 1985, the FDA approved the use of a biosynthetic replacement hormone for GH deficient children. Almost identical to pituitary GH, the new product was called *somatrem* to distinguish it from *somatotropin*, the natural stuff.

GH In Vivo and In Vitro

A milligram of GH sits idle in a petri dish. The shallow round piece of laboratory crockery with its loose fitting top is a place where biological processes can be studied on the small scale. Another way to say something was studied in a petri dish is *in vitro*, which means in glass, as opposed to *in vivo*, which means in the living body. Anyway, this milliliter of GH just sits there in the petri dish inert, looking hormone-like. In fact, under most circumstances, when researchers put GH *in vitro* with samples of body tissues, the dynamic hormone didn't do much of anything. Most of what is known about GH had to be discovered *in vivo*, as a part of the whole working system from hypothalamus to target organs and back again through feedback mechanisms.

Let's take it from the top.

The Hypothalamus: Go or No Go

The hypothalamus, an organ of the mid-brain, is the director of anterior pituitary secretions. The hypothalamus sends its chemical messages through the pituitary stalk. If you cut the pituitary stalk from the hypothalamus, the pituitary simply doesn't work and GH and other pituitary hormones are not produced. The substance that carries hypothalamic messages to the GH-producing cells in the anterior pituitary was first called *growth hormone releasing factor* (GH-RF or GRF), and when its nature was further understood, growth hormone releasing hormone (GHRH). The existence of this hormone or releasing factor was hypothesized for about twenty years before it could be isolated. When it was discovered in 1982, it was isolated not from tissues of the hypothalamus but from tumors of the pancreas. These abnormal cells were found to be producing a substance that increased GH flow and later was proved to be identical to hypothalamic GHRH. Synthesized by the ever active H.G. Li, biologic forms of this protein substance have been available for research purposes since the late 1980s but have not yet been approved for general clinical use by the FDA.

In an unsuccessful attempt in 1972 to isolate GHRH from crude hypothalamic extracts, researchers at the Salk Institute in La Jolla, California, discovered a substance that had exactly the opposite effect. The more of this new substance present, the less GH is secreted. The Salk researchers called the substance *somatotropin release inhibiting factor* or SRIF. The description of the newly discovered protein quickly led to its synthesis. Later researchers called the substance GH-IH or *growth hormone release inhibiting hormone*. Others named it *somatostatin*.

Using these two substances, the hypothalamus orders up more GH production from the pituitary or cancels the order. Which factor the hypothalamus sends depends a large part on messages from the feedback system which report current levels of the substances GH controls.

The Anterior Pituitary

If you look closely at a pituitary gland, you see a slight line that marks the juncture of the two lobes of the pituitary gland, the anterior pituitary and the posterior pituitary. The anterior pituitary can be distinguished from the posterior pituitary by its darker color caused by its more abundant blood supply.

The cells of the anterior pituitary all seem the same under the light microscope but, when they are stained with dye, five different kinds of cells can be distinguished by the way they absorb the dye. Each kind of cell normally secretes a certain trophic hormone. (*Thyrotrophs* secrete *thyrotropin, gonadotrophs* secrete *luteinizing hormone* and *follicle stimulating hormone, corticotrophs* secrete *adrenocorticotropic hormone, lactotrophs* secrete *prolactin*.) The cells that secrete *somatotropin* (growth hormone) are called *somatotrophs*. Somatotrophs in fact make up about 40% of the anterior pituitary.

The somatotrophs continuously manufacture GH, then, under the stimulation of GHRH, release the hormone in spurts, a total of one to two milligrams of GH per day.

Dream and Grow

You know the old saying that you grow while you sleep? It's more than a saying. In fact, the largest surge of GH hormone occurs one or two hours after you fall asleep; other surges occur during the night, primarily when you dream. Less dramatic ups and downs occur during the day, approximately every three hours. A larger surge is expected three to five hours after eating. See the graph below which represents a typical GH-release pattern for a normal young adult male.

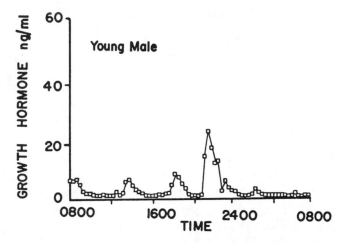

A representative GH profile from a young male sampled every 20 minutes for 24 hours. Pulses were categorized as large (L) or small (S) depending on whether the rise was greater or less than three times the threshold criterion for a pulse.

From Ho K.Y., Evans W.S., Blizzard R.M., Veldhuis J.D., Merriam G.R., Samojlik E., Furlanetto R., Rogol A.D., Kaiser D.L. and Thorner M.O., used with permission of The Edocrine Society from "Effects of Sex and Age on the 24-hour Profile of Growth Hormone Secretion in Man," Journal of Clinical Endocrinology and Metabolism, *1987; vol. 64, pp. 51-57.*

In addition, a jolt of GH is stimulated both by that popular cure-all—exercise—and by that old bugaboo—stress. The variable release of GH throughout the day makes comparative measurement of GH difficult.

Receptors

GH, circulating around the body in the bloodstream, would not be able to deliver its growth messages if something at the target organ didn't recognize the messenger and sign for the package. Body tissues do not respond to a hormone if they do not possess receptors for that hormone. What complicates the delivery is that different classes of receptors are looking for different messages associated with distinctive GH action. It's only through examining the receptors that we begin to understand the many actions of GH.

One means of identifying receptors is through *radio receptor assay*. Some of the hormone is labeled in a laboratory with radioactive Iodogen to serve as a tracer. The iodinated GH (I-hGH), injected into the bloodstream, will achieve as much as 85% binding on various target cells, as indicated by the location of the radioactive material.

You might think the major receptors would be on skeletal cells, since skeletal growth is the hallmark of GH action. Not so, for reasons to be explained later. In fact, the liver has been found to be the major target organ. GH receptors have been found at many other sites from mammary glands to fat tissue.

GH binds to specific receptor sites on the surface of target cell membranes. Substances antagonistic to GH (dopamine, for example) compete for binding space on receptor cells and in this way may serve as regulators.

Indirect Action of GH

From a substance called growth hormone, what you expect is growth. Accordingly, researchers Salmon and Daughaday in 1957 put GH in petri dishes with animal cartilage samples and waited for them to grow. Nothing. But the cells of the same cartilage in the presence of blood serum from an animal with plenty of circulating GH multiplied. Why would GH-rich blood but not GH itself stimulate growth activity? The research team from Washington University concluded the growth-promoting action of GH was indirect. There must be something else in the blood that mediated the GH action. They called this intermediary the *sulfation factor* since the uptake and incorporation of sulfate is an essential indication of tissue growth. The sulfation factor was soon understood to be more than one, and they were renamed the *somatomedins*.

Three somatomedins were named somatomedin A, B, and C. In the meantime, another team of investigators discovered a substance the same as somatomedin-C (Sm-C) and, not knowing it was the same, named it *insulinlike growth factor-I* (IGF-I). Although many people are accustomed to using the word *somatomedin-C*, researchers on the cutting edge prefer *IGF-I* because of the substance's relationship to IGF-II, which is not a somatomedin. Some researchers use the term Sm-C/IGF-I (and also IGF-I/Sm-C) to resolve the issue. S-M-C-I-G-F-I doesn't exactly slide off the tongue—or the finger on the keyboard—but we will use the term anyway (although we privately pronounce it "Smurf-One"). Remember the substance Sm-C/IGF-I any way you can because it's important. (You can pronounce it "Smurf-One," also, if it helps, but don't tell anyone you heard it from us.)

Sm-C/IGF-I is produced largely in the main GH-target organ—the liver—but it can be produced by many other kinds of cells. Sm-C/IGF-I, in turn, moves on to its own specialized target organs with their specialized receptors.

Cartilage cells make up an important target for Sm-

C/IGF-I. Under the influence of Sm-C/IGF-I, cartilage cells proliferate, ultimately hardening into bone. Skeletal growth is therefore a *direct* action of Sm-C/IGF-I and an *indirect* action of GH.

GH, through Sm-C/IGF-I, also causes an increase in the number and size of muscle cells and a shift to a positive nitrogen balance. This explains why children treated with GH to increase their height become more muscular, and this is why elderly people like those Rudman studied reclaim some of the muscle of their youth when GH is restored. In fact, Sm-C/IGF-I was the substance Rudman measured as a means of assessing circulating GH levels in his elderly male subjects instead of testing them for GH directly.

Direct Effects of GH

In addition to the indirect action of GH through Sm-C/IGF-I, there are important direct effects of the growth hormone. Direct effects of GH include the breaking down of fats into free fatty acids. As Judson J. Van Wyk and colleagues at the University of North Carolina School of Medicine have noted, "Hypopituitary children have stores of ripply fat that melt away with GH administration" as did the fat of Rudman's elderly male subjects. The fat-busting provides energy for the growth that is stimulated. The stimulation of a variety of enzymes in the liver is another direct effect of GH. The combined effect of cortisol—a hormone of the adrenal cortex—and GH in the regulation of blood sugar is a third direct effect of GH that requires no intermediary hormone.

The Imperfect Dichotomy

It has been observed that under certain circumstances GH shares *some* of the same metabolic pathways as insulin, the sugar metabolizing hormone made in the pancreas; under other circumstances GH acts in opposition to insulin. The insulinlike and non-insulinlike categories of action correspond roughly with the direct and indirect action of GH.

The dichotomy of direct and indirect action of GH is an over-simplification in which the divvying up has not gone unchallenged. In what we call the Bugs Bunny Challenge, the idea that all cartilage growth is an indirect activity of GH was contradicted. In that study a form of GH did directly stimulate growth related processes in cultured cartilage cells from a rabbit ear. There was also a Rat Rib Challenge and a Monkey Paw Challenge, which also belied the indirect action model. Whether GH acts directly or indirectly on growing tissues is still very much open to investigation with growing evidence that part of the process is direct and part is indirect.

Also, while GH receptors are predominantly in the liver, they have also been found all over the body; it is not known how GH works in these cells. What's more, some things happen around GH that neither the direct or indirect theories can explain. New hypotheses under investigation are likely to complicate as well as clarify the picture of GH action.

Checks and Balances:
The Autofeedback System

The release of GH is pulsatile, its ebb and flow corresponding to the stimulation of GHRH (GH releasing hormone) and the inhibition of somatostatin (GH inhibiting factor or GRIF). This go/no-go pattern in the hypothalamus is in turn critically influenced by the blood levels of GH itself. Thus when GHRH gives the green light to the pituitary to release GH, the surge of

GH goes to receptor sites all around the body *and* back to the hypothalamus to say, "Hey, it worked. You can take it easy now."

In peripheral tissues, the long-acting cascade effects of Sm-C/IGF-I smooth out the episodic events at the hypothalamic/pituitary level. The level of Sm-C/IGF-I in the blood also contributes information to the hypothalamus and pituitary and is a major player, sometimes the overriding force, in the feedback system.

In what is known as an Ultrashort Feedback Loop, somatostatin may inhibit GHRH release directly and GHRH may stimulate the release of somatostatin. Like two evenly matched opponents neither lets the other get the upper hand.

To complicate matters, somatostatin is secreted not only in the hypothalamus but also in various parts of the central nervous system, in the spinal cord and the beta cells of the entire GI tract and undoubtedly plays a part is GH regulation.

When all is working well, the feedback system seems unessential to understanding GH. However, in unusual cases like disease or treatment of children with GH by injection, what happens to the feedback system can be critical.

In a Nutshell

GH made in the pituitary is released under the influence of releasing and inhibiting hormones from the hypothalamus. It travels all over the body acting directly on organs through receptor cells or indirectly through somatomedin-C/insulinlike growth factor-I. Sm-C/IGF-I, made in the liver and other tissues, acts on cartilage cells at the bone growth plates to cause skeletal growth. Equally important as skeletal growth is GH's effects on body composition. GH, released es-

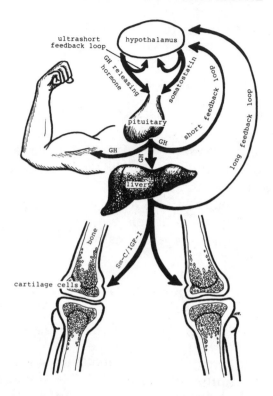

THE PATH OF GROWTH HORMONE ACTION

Stimulating and inhibiting hormones from the hypothalamus direct the release of GH from the pituitary. GH has direct action on many peripheral tissues. The major target organ of GH is the liver. The liver produces Sm-C/IGF-I which, in turn, acts on the cartilage cells of the bone to promote growth. At each stage, hormone levels act as feedback mechanisms to the hypothalamus. *Illustration by Nathan McKnight.*

pecially in times of increased activity, stress, and famine, acts to conserve muscle tissue at the expense of fat tissues—a function which favored the survival of primitive man and helps today's flabbier folks hold onto a lean and hungry look a little longer.

Too Much of a Good Thing

If Growth Hormone is so great, wouldn't more GH be even better? That question certainly arose in the mind of the public who read about the findings of the Rudman study. Can you benefit from GH even if you are not GH deficient? And, if some GH therapy recaptured some tissue "youth," would more GH recapture even more youth? Can there be too much of a good thing?

The answer to the last question is certainly Yes. Too much GH in the system can produce dramatic disorders. One of them is *gigantism*, also called *giantism*, which can affect children, adolescents, and others whose open growth plates allow the bones to continue to lengthen. (See illustration on the next page.) Excess GH in adults and others whose growth plates have closed is called *acromegaly*. Both are rare and interesting disorders that have provided many clues to the normal role of growth hormone.

Giants: The Big Picture

David slew one giant named Goliath, Jack faced one

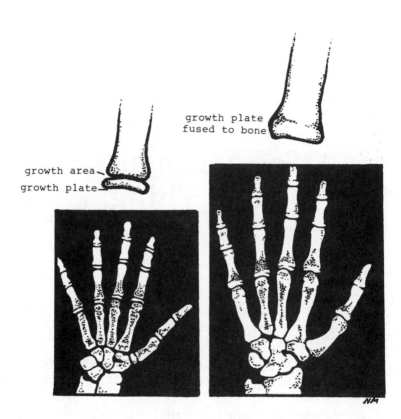

growth plate
fused to bone

growth area
growth plate

Hand Bones of a Young Child
Growth plates at the ends of
bone cap areas of cartilage
cells where growth occurs.
Illustrations by Nathan McKnight.

Hand Bones of a Late Adolescent
Growth plates are almost completely fused to the bone so
that further growth in bone
length cannot occur.

at the top of the beanstalk, and another was the greatest
lumberjack of all. The giant of myth and legend was
sometimes a fictional character who met the storytell-
ers' need for the superlative. Often, however, the giant
was very real. His physical attributes may have been
exaggerated in the telling, but the dramatic effect of

standing head and shoulders above the crowd was true to life.

Greek historian Herodotus, a contemporary of Hippocrates, described a man 5 royal cubits tall, that is, 8 feet 2 inches, who "had the loudest voice in the world." After the battle of Plataea in 479 B.C, Medvei tells us, a body found among the Persian dead measured 7 feet 6 inches. These giants were real.

In the biblical story of David and Goliath of Gath, the champion of the Philistines stood "six cubits and a span." This measure translated into the unlikely height of 9 feet 6 1/2 inches. But early Greek translations of the Old Testament as well as an account by a Hebrew historian born in the first century A.D. credits Goliath with the more believable height of four Greek cubits and a span, or 6 feet 10 inches. That put the Philistine hero well into the giant category in his day, towering above his fellow soldiers. The fact that David made short work of Goliath, planting a stone from his slingshot into the giant's forehead, is not inconsistent with gigantism. Real life giants are not necessarily tough. Their strength depends on what kind of giant they are.

There are pituitary giants that have too much GH, usually because of a tumor in the anterior pituitary, and there are familial giants, that is, those who are born to very tall parents. The most common reason for being very tall has always been having a very tall parent. In addition, tall people tend to marry tall people, and the children of two tall parents have an even higher probability of inheriting genes for tallness.

Genetic factors account for the over-six-feet average height of males of the Watusi tribe of Central Africa and of the equally statuesque Dinka tribe in the Sudan. A 6-feet-3-inch Watusi would be just one of the guys. A

6-feet-3-inch pygmy, however, would be a giant. Gigantism is relative.

Goliath was relatively giant. But did he have an overactive pituitary causing excess growth hormone? Probably not.

Medvei has done some giant genealogy and tells us that Goliath was probably descended from the remnants of a tribe of giants that took refuge with the Philistines after being driven out of their own land by conquering Ammonites. "That also was accounted a land of giants: giants dwelt therein in old time." (Deuteronomy, ii, 20) In a series of battles several years after the David and Goliath match, (Samuel II, xxi, 15-22), David and the forces of Israel faced four more giants fighting on the side of the Philistines. This time David himself was a little faint, but his soldiers slew all four giants, described as "sons of the giant" and "born to the giant of Gath." If Goliath was descended from giants and fathered four giants, his gianthood was obviously inherited. By contrast, pituitary giants tend to be impotent and sterile and incapable of passing on their traits. Besides, far from being mighty warriors, they tend to be weak, bearing with difficulty the weight of their overgrown bones.

The same criteria can be applied to the Norse tribes who once roamed Greenland, giants from the Fyrdafjord district of Norway, or huge sea raiders depicted in rock tracings of southern Sweden. If these oversized people were suffering from the disorder of pituitary gigantism, that is, too much GH, they were unlikely to be strong enough to plunder and sail the seas.

No research has indicated a direct connection between familial height and degree of pituitary activity. Normal tall people do not have more GH; normal short people do not have less GH. The most recent explanation for inherited tall stature is that families of normally tall people and whole tribes of tall people share an inherited characteristic, namely, that their GH receptors are more sensitive to GH than the receptors of other families or other tribes. The connection between excess GH and extreme height—gigantism—remains in the domain of the abnormal.

When, in the nineteenth century, scientists finally connected the pituitary with growth, they became eager to examine the remains of giants for clues to their bizarre condition. According to Medvei, one was Irish giant Cornelius Magrath, who at age sixteen was a shade under 6-feet 9 inches and still growing. Befriended in the 1750s by the Bishop of Cloyne, Magrath was thought by his countrymen to be a product of the Bishop's "experiments in giant-rearing." Magrath's skull was available for study in the nineteenth century and was the subject of an 1891 monograph which described the enlarged sella turcica where a pituitary tumor the size of a small tangerine must have been growing.

Experimental anatomist John Hunter bought the skeleton of another eighteenth-century Irish giant, Charles Byrne, for the fine sum of 500 British pounds to put in his museum of specimens. From the distended sella turcica it was concluded that Byrne also suffered from an enlarged pituitary or tumor. Drawing from such evidence, scientists began to connect the condition of gigantism with an overgrown pituitary. They did not yet understand that the enlarged gland produced excessive quantities of hormones.

The widow of another giant, Sieur Mirbeck, refused to allow an autopsy of her husband before burying him with dignity. Nevertheless, three years later, under mysterious circumstances, the breastbone, left collarbone, and a right rib of the deceased were obtained from the grave and sold to the museum of another celebrated endocrinologist. Rarity was the key to the celebrity of the bones of giants.

"Pituitary growth hormone excess is a rare cause of excessive growth during childhood or adolescence," says John S. Parks, M.D., of the Emory University School of Medicine. "However, it is thought to account for more than half of the instances of adult heights over seven feet."

According to Guinness

The tallest medically verified man on record, Robert Wadlaw, passed the 8-feet mark at eighteen years of age, according to the *Guinness Book of World Records*. But he didn't quit there. He continued to grow to a height of 8 feet 11 inches. He was a hefty but normal 8 1/2 pounds at his birth in 1918, but his growth took off at about age two. Wadlaw's gigantism, like that of other eight-footers, was a combination of fast growth due to excess GH and a failure of the bone growth plates to close at a normal age. Although the Illinois native ate about 8,000 calories a day, and his highest weight was 490 pounds, he was never anything but slender. With a size 37 AA shoe, foot-long hand, and 9-feet-5 3/4-inch arm span, it took a lot of nourishment to keep him going.

The tallest woman in history was Zeng Jinlian of Hunan, China, who grew to be 8-feet 1 3/4 inches. She could not stand erect by the time she died in 1982.

The tallest living woman is a resident of Shelbyville, Indiana. Sandy Allen weighed a mere 6 1/2 pounds at birth; her rapid growth started soon afterwards. By the age of 22 she was 7-feet 7 1/4 inches. At that point she had pituitary surgery to halt the excess production of

GH. A picture in the 1988 *Guinness Book of World Records* shows Sandy towering over her normal-sized friends and wearing a big smile and a T-shirt asking the rest of the world, "How'd you get so short?" A smile and a sense of humor go a long way to make gigantism bearable.

Other American giants listed in the *Guinness Book of World Records* are 8-feet-8-inch John William Rogan (1871-1905) of Gallatin, Tennessee, who was still growing at the time of his death. Don Koehler, a Montana native, hit an abnormal growth spurt beginning at age ten which took him to a height of 8-feet 2 inches. Koehler, who died in 1981 at the age of 56, lived the longest of any of the eight-footers listed by Guinness.

Vaino Myllyrinne (1909-1963) of Helsinki, Finland, stood over 7 feet 3 inches at age twenty-one and seemed to be settling down at that height, but in his late thirties he had a growth spurt that took him to 8 feet 3 inches. Gabriele Mojane, born in 1944 in Mozambique, measured 7 feet 10 inches at the age of twenty-one. He was estimated to be just over 8 feet at his death in 1990, although as a circus attraction he was billed at 8 feet 3 inches. It is customary for circuses to exaggerate the proportions of its giants and dwarfs and to write into the contract that actual measurement will not be allowed.

This spectacle is interesting but sad. There is no reason whatsoever that a pituitary giant's growth could not be stopped by treatment. The benefits of celebrity never outweigh the problems associated with gigantism.

Pituitary gigantism can be devastating. Robert Wadlaw had to wear a brace on his ankle. His rapid growth had also limited the feeling in his legs. Consequently, he did not feel a blister caused by the rubbing of the brace. An infection of that blister ultimately resulted in his death at the age of twenty-two. Of the nine other men over 8 feet tall listed in the *Guinness Book of World Records*, one had severe kypho-scoliosis (two-dimensional spinal curvature), one was measured in a sitting position because his joints were so stiff he could not stand, and one had both legs amputated because of gangrene.

Even people whose gigantism is less dramatic fare poorly. A recent study of pituitary giants living in London indicated that practically all were handicapped by kypho-scoliosis and other complications and that all led reclusive lives.

An American seven-footer observes:"I never go anywhere that people don't stare. And no one can talk to me face to face standing up. Some people try. They talk politely for a few seconds and then they go away. They can't go on craning their neck and I can't be bobbing up and down so we can hear each other. Conversation is impossible except sitting down. Not too many people want to sit down with me. It's hard for me to get to that point. Yes, I'd like to be normal sized and have people interested in *me*, not just my oddity."

When Is Tall Too Tall?

While the medical definition of gigantism suggests an underlying pathology, the practical diagnosis relies heavily on measuring and comparing. According to Parks, one of the nation's foremost pediatric endocrinologists, gigantism or "excessive growth is defined as a process leading to stature above the range appropriate for a child or adolescent's age, sex, and genetic background." The diagnosis of gigantism must occur during the childhood period if any intervention in growth is expected.

The tools for assessing growth are a ruler for measuring height, a scale, and a set of age and sex-appropriate growth charts designed by the National Center for Health Statistics (NCHS).

The charts on the following pages are a NCHS chart for boys between the ages of two and eighteen. The boys' chart, like the corresponding girls' chart, shows height on the vertical lines and age on the horizontal lines. The height of 90% of all boys will fall between the top curved line and the bottom curved line across the chart. Any boy whose height lies above the top curve is exceptionally tall, but not necessarily abnormal. Normally a boy's growth will follow the curve, near the top if he will be tall, near the middle if he will be average, near the bottom if he will be short.

Birth weight has little to do with eventual height, but usually by the age of two a child settles into a channel—the space between two of the percentile curves on the chart—according to his genetic makeup—and he follows that curve rather closely until maturity. The first chart shows a normal tall boy growing through the years to become a normal tall adult. The second chart shows a boy who was growing near the average curve until about age eight. At this point his growth began to rise rapidly above the channel he was in. His growth curve crossed two channels in two years. Such a child is experiencing a rapid growth spurt that may indicate abnormal development.

Parks says, "Criteria for growth excess include a height above the 99th percentile for age and sex, a height more than three channels above the mid-parental height, or a crossing of more than two channels after two years of age.

"Family history of pace and timing of puberty is also important," says Parks. "The tall child may be express-

BOYS FROM 2 TO 18 YEARS
STATURE FOR AGE

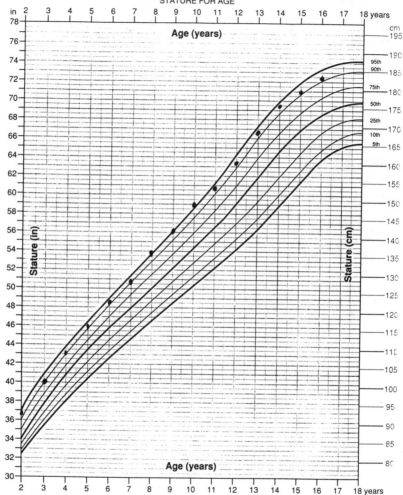

Height Measurements of a Normal Tall Boy

Normal growth marks form a steadily rising curve over time.
Norms from National Center for Health Statistics, chart distributed by Mead Johnson Nutritionals.

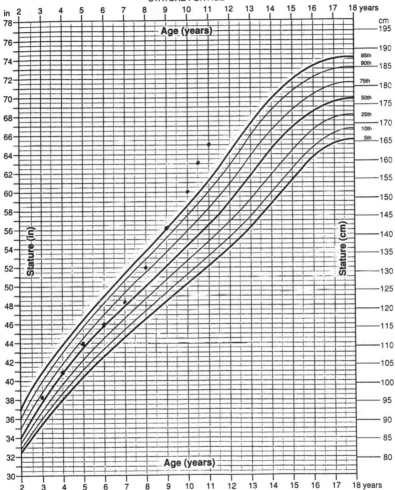

BOYS FROM 2 TO 18 YEARS
STATURE FOR AGE

Height Measurements of an Abnormally Rapid Growth Spurt

Height that crosses two channels after the age of two years should be evaluated. *Norms from National Center for Health Statistics, chart distributed by Mead Johnson Nutritionals.*

ing a familial tendency for early maturation rather than for tall adult stature." Ginny, for instance, was 5 feet 5 inches at the age of ten. Towering above her peers she felt like a giant. In those days, no one thought of medical intervention, and, as usually happened, none was necessary. Within the year she matured physically and stopped growing. Soon she found herself right in the average range of her friends.

When Ginny had a daughter who was even taller than she had been at age ten, she was uneasy because she remembered her own feelings of insecurity as a tall child. She consulted her pediatrician. A quick interview revealed Ginny's own history, and she was reassured that time would take care of the problem, which it did.

Even when children are surely headed for extreme height, few suffer from medically defined gigantism. Parents, however, often have a different and subjective criteria for acceptable height, especially for girls.

In the 1960s, four brothers, all over 6 feet 6 inches, played on two state championship basketball teams during their combined high school playing years. They enjoyed immensely their status as local heros. Later they all played college ball, setting several ACC records. One went on to play pro ball; another, at 6 feet 8 inches, was turned down in a military draft for meeting the military definition of a giant—anyone over 6 feet 6 inches.

The brothers all married girls about 5 feet 6 inches and raised larger than average children. Several of the boys nearly reached their fathers' heights as teenagers and headed for the basketball court. Fine. When one of the daughters was 5 feet 9 1/2 inches at age thirteen, however, her parents took her to an endocrinologist. It was never a question of a disorder. Parents and physicians recognized the natural playing out of the genes. But the girl was too tall!

The girl's mother, Robin, a beautiful 5 feet 6 inches, recalls having reached her adult height as early as the fifth grade. "I felt like there was too much of me. I could never be cute like other girls. When my mother took me to buy a dress, the salesclerk would say to my mother, 'My, she's a healthy girl.' She didn't mean I was free of disease; she meant I was too big to fit into dresses appropriate for my age."

Robin's daughter, 22 inches at birth, was always thereafter above the 95th channel on the growth chart. Robin noticed that preschool teachers would tell her child to give up a desired toy and "let the little ones have it." She was treated as an older child, expected to humor the younger ones.

Because of her sensitivity to the issue of height, Robin took her daughter to an endocrinologist before the daughter had complained of being too tall. Endocrinologists gave the girl hormones to shorten her adolescent growth spurt and bring her to maturity before she had reached her natural genetic height. Some people would criticize, saying that Robin, in seeking treatment for the daughter, was acting out of her own needs rather than supporting her daughter's satisfaction with her size, but Robin feels justified. In a couple years the teenager, who stopped growing at 5 feet 11 inches, expressed gratitude that she was not any taller. Also, a moderate scoliosis that resisted treatment is probably less troublesome at her current height than her projected height of well over 6 feet.

Some other girls in tall families, of course, think nothing of their exceptional height, carry it well, and enjoy the distinction.

Familial tall stature, seen especially on the basketball

court, does not come from greater-than-average GH secretion, but may involve an inherited greater-than-average responsiveness of receptors to GH.

Other Kinds of Giants

There are several causes of gigantism, only one of them having to do with excessive growth hormone. It is useful to note the others and distinguish them from those with a pituitary disorder.

First, there are several genetic diseases marked by growth excess during childhood. *Marfan Syndrome*, a disease of the connective tissue, results in tall stature with unusually long bones and fingers. Other abnormalities may include weakness in joints and blood vessels and scoliosis, but many people with the disease appear healthy. Sooner or later an aortic aneurysm (a ballooning out of the wall of the major blood vessel leading out of the heart), which is characteristic of the syndrome, may burst during physical exertion. Undetected Marfan Syndrome accounts for the death of Flo Hyman, charismatic American volleyball star, during a match in Japan in 1986. She had felt self-conscious about being 6 feet tall in elementary school but her adult height of six feet 5 inches served the 1984 Olympian well on the court. After her death, Hyman's siblings, all tall, were tested for the disease, which affects about 40,000 Americans. One brother tested positive and had corrective heart surgery. Some experts think Abraham Lincoln, unusually tall for his day and often described as "gangly," may have had Marfan's Syndrome. Recently, the National Museum of Health and Medicine, which holds some tissues from Abraham Lincoln's body—blood stains on his physician's shirtsleeve, to be exact—began laying the ground work for testing the DNA of the sixteenth president for Marfan

Syndrome. The instigators of this investigation hope that, if the tests are positive, the revelation will create more public awareness of the disease.

Cerebral gigantism or *Soto's Syndrome* is also genetic. At birth, the baby is heavy as well as long and develops disproportionately long hands and feet and coarse facial features. *Beckwith-Wiedemann Syndrome* often involves the enlargement of certain internal organs and unusual ear creases. Some children with this syndrome have been found to have a chromosome abnormality which may affect the genes for insulin and insulinlike growth factor II. Two other rare genetic diseases causing abnormal growth in children, *Klinefelter Syndrome* and *XYY Chromosome Syndrome*, may be accompanied by learning disabilities. These genetic syndromes are picked up by doctors more readily from the associated symptoms than from the excess height.

Another whole category of gigantism has to do with hormonal overproduction. Hyperthyroidism, excess production of thyroid hormone, will make children large for their age. Since skeletal maturity is also advanced, there is an early closure of growth plates or *epiphyses* at the ends of the long bones. Growth, therefore, stops before extreme gigantism occurs. An excess of the hormone insulin, a disorder of the pancreas, may also create excessively rapid growth in height along with obesity.

Gigantism in children as a result of too much sex hormone is a complicated issue. The child suffering from too much of various sex hormones secondary to an overactive adrenal gland or adrenal tumor will come to maturity too early. The adolescent growth spurt will also come much earlier. The child will therefore be too large for his age early on, but, by the time his peers mature, he will be no taller than expected from his parents' size, probably shorter. In some families, however, early puberty is an inherited trait and can be recognized from a family history.

Gigantism as a result of excess growth hormone is actually one of the rarest types and is suspected only when other factors are ruled out. Physicians interviewed in several pediatric endocrinology departments at major medical schools said they had seen only one or two cases of juvenile growth hormone gigantism in their careers. One physician had seen a single case, a young girl in the 95th percentile of height for her age. He recalls being approached by the girl's father who had concluded the girl was secreting too much growth hormone. The doctor, however, took a look at the father, who was well above average in height himself, and concluded the daughter was just a long sliver off the old block. The father insisted on having his daughter tested for GH anyway. To the doctor's surprise, she tested high. Further investigation revealed the cause—a small GH-secreting pituitary tumor which was successfully removed. The girl in this case was lucky to achieve early diagnosis before other kinds of damage from the tumor appeared.

Again, we must note that this rare juvenile patient was a girl. People are quick to see tall stature in a girl as something wrong. When a very young girl begins to come up to her father's chin, her parents take her to a doctor. When a boy, on the other hand, seems headed for the sky, parents send him to the basketball coach. Because tallness is considered an asset for boys, extremely rapid growth is often not recognized as a disorder unless other abnormal symptoms appear.

When children reach puberty, the growth plates have closed, the bones will not be extended by the indirect action of growth hormone. Growth hormone continues to have a role in bone remodeling and tissue growth and repair, but its bone lengthening days are over. If, however, a pituitary tumor exists and the overproduction of GH continues, the effects of that overgrowth will be seen in a disorder called *acromegaly*.

Acromegaly: Growing Out Instead of Up

Dr. James H. Christy, an endocrinologist at the Emory University Clinic, looked down the hall and saw a couple walking towards him. He knew right away who his next patient would be even though he had not looked at the chart. The man, accompanied by his wife, was an acromegalic, that is, he suffered the effects of too much growth hormone. "When you've seen as many acromegalics as I have you know it by a glance at their face," says Dr. Christy. The man had coarse features—large lips, a very long nose with enlarged nostrils, and a bulging forehead.

The man strode up to the doctor and offered his large spade-like hand which Dr. Christy shook firmly. "Steve _____," the man introduced himself. When Steve, his wife, and the physician were comfortably seated in his office, Dr. Christy looked earnestly at Steve and said, "Now how long have you had this condition?"

"No, Doctor Christy, it's not me. It's my wife. Our family doctor says she has a problem with her thyroid gland."

Dr. Christy was startled. A glance at the chart his nurse had laid out confirmed that the appointment was for the wife.

"You may not be my patient, but you are someone's patient," Dr. Christy said to Steve. "You used to wear a wedding ring?"

"Yes, but it got too small for my finger."

"No, your finger got too large for the ring. What size shoe do you wear?"

"Twelve."

"And what size did you wear before?"

"Come to think of it, I used to wear a ten."

"How long ago was that?"

"About two years ago."

"That's how long you have had a tumor on your pituitary gland," said Dr. Christy.

The physician explained that Steve had too much growth hormone in his blood. The GH was causing the bones and cartilage to grow most noticeably in his face and hands and feet. Dr. Christy knew that the excess GH was not a condition present before puberty because the man was a normal 6 feet in height. If he had had too much GH as a child when his growth plates were open for growth, he would have grown far above normal size. He almost certainly had a tumor of recent origin on his pituitary gland that was causing it to produce too much growth hormone. Such tumors are rarely malignant and almost always treatable.

"Do you have diabetes?"

Steve looked really surprised. "How did you know? I have been treated by eight doctors and they all say I will be diabetic for the rest of my life."

"I can cure that, if you'll let me," said Dr. Christy. "You have the only kind of diabetes that can be cured."

GH is an antagonist to insulin. In too large quantities, GH makes the system resistant to insulin, the hormone that metabolizes sugar. GH excess in many cases thereby causes diabetes.

"Did you notice that your husband's looks were changing?" Dr. Christy asked Steve's wife.

"No. But now that you point it out, I realize that he

has changed. I just thought it was because he was getting older." Steve was 36.

Once diagnosed, Steve began to realize that a number of other problems that had seemed unrelated were actually the result of acromegaly. He was sleepy all the time, perhaps from the diabetes. The cartilage changes in his nose had caused him to snore so loudly, his wife was at the end of her rope. He couldn't get gloves to fit and wondered why manufacturers made size large so small. Even his hairs were growing so big around that they felt stiff to the touch. But these changes had not seemed to him to be the sort of things he should bring up to a doctor treating diabetes.

Dr. Christy's diagnosis of excessive GH secretion was confirmed by a series of hormone studies, including a growth hormone assay. Soon afterwards Steve went for an MRI (magnetic resonance imaging). In the imaging clinic, he was moved, lying down, into a cylinder that was so small in diameter that he decided to close his eyes, fearing he would panic in such a tight place. (Severe claustrophobics are given the option of a CT scan which does not involve being confined but produces pictures with less clear resolution.) Steve could hear his wife and her mother talking outside the cylinder but he did not feel like saying much himself. Then the pounding began. It sounded as if someone were beating a drum and he was inside. The noise, as the machine worked, went on for an hour. Only when technicians were pulling Steve out of the cylinder did he dare open his eyes, curious to see what the interior looked like.

He was more pleased with the looks of the images. "They were so sharp, amazing. I could see my brain with all those wrinkles like they say you have, and I thought, now I know I really do have a brain." He also saw his pituitary gland and the tumor and the route the surgeon would take. It would begin just in front of his front teeth and under his lip and proceed up into the sphenoid sinus to the sella turcica where the tumor would be removed with the aid of a microscope.

The surgery, Steve said, was not so bad. Of course, he was asleep. When it was finished, it only required one stitch. What bothered Steve the most was the incision on his abdomen where the surgeon cut off a piece of fat to plug various holes made on the way up to the pituitary.

"It was certainly worth it," says Steve. Tests showed his abnormal growth hormone secretion immediately dropped off after surgery. The size of his hands decreased just as quickly and his wife soon could see a difference in his face as soft tissue shrank. To Dr. Christy's highly trained eye, Steve still has the look of a treated acromegalic because he retains some bony prominence and extra cartilage, but to most of us he seems like a good looking guy with a rather big nose, somewhere between Durante's and Cyranno's. "I'm thankful I was treated before it got any worse," he says.

The main improvement was in how Steve felt. He got his old energy back and his diabetes was resolved. He no longer faces the health risks of either acromegaly or diabetes. Monitoring indicates that Steve's healthy pituitary is now making normal amounts of GH and of other anterior pituitary hormones as well.

Those of you who have not forgotten about Steve's wife's thyroid problem will be happy to know that Dr. Christy successfully treated her, too.

The Case of the Moving Teeth

At the age of 40, William J. concluded something was seriously wrong. His lower teeth no longer met his upper teeth in the way they had, and he had gone from an overbite to an underbite. When his dentist confirmed this degree of change was abnormal, acromegaly was the number one suspect; the lower jaw is known to be particularly sensitive to GH excess.

The pituitary tumor found to be causing William's excessive GH production was successfully removed through surgery. Afterwards, his teeth did not move back in place because bone and cartilage growth is permanent, but William says, "The operation was worth it just for the way I could breathe again. I couldn't believe what a relief it was." Excess tissue in his nasal passages had caused him a great deal of trouble, but never having heard of acromegaly, he could not relate that problem to the changes in his jaw, the increase of his ring size from 12 to 20, and border-line diabetes.

Since his experience, William, a retired manufacturing plant manager, has spotted and informed two other acromegalics. One lived in William's boyhood community. "We dated the same girl way back when," he recalls. William got the fellow to a doctor but it was too late. The tumor could not be completely excised and the man died about ten years later at the age of fifty, still suffering from some of the effects of the disease. More recently, William saw a man in an airport with by-now familiar symptoms of acromegaly. William approached him, also. The man was grateful, saying he knew something was going on but didn't know what; he promised to seek medical help. William never got the man's name and only hopes his case came to as successful conclusion as his own.

Not all diagnoses go so smoothly. In 1989 Dr. D. had a new patient come in for a routine exam. Dr. D., a general practitioner, had never treated an acromegalic in his entire practice, but he recognized the disease in his new patient immediately. When he explained the disease and pointed out its signs, the patient denied they were anything unusual. His protruding jaw? A simple malocclusion that had always been there. The bulging brow? From his mother's side of the family. The spade hands? His brothers all had large hands like that.

Other than the enlarged tissue, Dr. D. was unable to turn up any evidence of acromegaly to convince the patient. There was no sign of diabetes, no headaches or visual disturbance to indicate the presumed pituitary tumor. Dr. D. urged the patient to go get an MRI to see if there was a tumor anyway and warned him to look for other symptoms of acromegaly. The patient went away unconvinced and untreated.

About a year later, however, Dr. D. received an inquiry from an eye doctor about that same patient. The man was now having trouble with his peripheral vision and had sought treatment for his eyes. As it turned out, the pituitary tumor whose existence Dr. D. had suspected had grown upward and was pressing on the optic chiasm, causing abnormalities of the visual field. The correct treatment was, of course, the removal of the pituitary tumor. When the surgery had been done, the man's vision returned to normal and his abnormally enlarged soft tissue shrank; the protruding jaw, bony brow, and spade hands remained—but then, these "ran in the family."

While acromegaly is often slow or intermittent in developing and may not cause serious problems in a lifetime, untreated acromegaly can also be very harmful. Distortions hidden inside the body are less noticeable but more dangerous than the flesh, bone and cartilage distortions apparent from the outside.

In acromegaly, not only the hands, feet, and facial features but most organs become enlarged. An enlarged larynx (voice box) and nasal sinus gives an unusually resonant, deep, loud voice like the one Herodotus described as "the loudest voice in the world." A space may develop between the teeth as the jawbone enlarges. Not only do the ridges above the eyes enlarge, increasing the slope of the forehead, but the skin thickens and on the brow a skin fold becomes a permanent furrow or scowl. The liver, spleen, kidney, pancreas, and heart enlarge.

These changes are accompanied by a disturbance in functioning so severe that half of all untreated acromegalics die by age 50 and 89% die by age 60 from complications. One in three acromegalics have high blood pressure. Cardiac failure occurs in about a fourth, and a half develop sugar intolerance or full-blown diabetes.

In some acromegalics other endocrine glands under the influence of the pituitary (the thyroid and the adrenal cortex) enlarge because the tumor may oversecrete other pituitary trophic hormones; these same glands may become *hypo*active later if the tumor presses enough on the pituitary gland to destroy to some degree its production of other trophic hormones. For example, the eventual loss of sexual function (impotence or cessation of ovulation and menstruation) often found in acromegalics may be a result of destruction of gonadotrophs.

Hyper-secretion of prolactin, common in acromegaly, may be another reason for decreased sexual function, since prolactin is antagonistic to gonad function. (Remember that prolactin's important job of stimulating milk production inhibits ovulation and pregnancy in a woman for a while after giving birth.)

Prolactin, similar to GH in structure and action, is sometimes secreted by the same tumor. In rare cases, a small percentage of acromegalics, both male and female, experience breast enlargement and even milk production because of the parallel over-secretion of prolactin.

In most cases of acromegaly, greatly increased sweating is also noted. The pituitary tumor pressing on overlying membranes causes headaches in a majority of acromegalics. If the abnormal tissue grows upward to press on the optic chiasm, abnormalities of the visual field occur.

Acromegalics, like giants, are prone to scoliosis and other skeletal deformities, and while strong and vigorous at the onset of the disease, may become weak as it progresses. Arthritis is a frequent complication and swelling of soft tissue in the hands often causes carpal tunnel syndrome, an inflammation of the wrists more often caused by using the computer keyboard too long. Acromegalics, while "overgrown," are not obese because GH breaks down peripheral fat using it as a source of energy for the growth of other tissue.

Unfortunately, many acromegalics seek treatment after much damage has been done. Dr. John Ward, professor emeritus of Emory University School of Medicine, recalls a young man of 35 who came into his office. "He had refused diagnosis. He was the most advanced case of acromegaly I had ever seen." The man had a large jaw with extreme malocclusion, an enormous brow, a large nose, thickened skin. He lost consciousness in Dr. Ward's office as he began to hemorrhage because of the tumor. Ward called for emergency surgery and the patient responded.

This patient had previously had one ring cut off because his enlarged finger became uncomfortable, but a second, larger ring was still on his hand. After recovering from the surgery, the young man returned to Ward's office. He was drumming his fingers on Ward's desk when the second ring fell off. The soft tissue on his fingers had returned to its normal size when his GH reached normal levels. Unfortunately, the once nice looking fellow had to live with the abnormal bony tissue.

Acromegaly is so rare, and so few people know about it, that self-diagnosis almost never occurs. Changes are gradual, and people who may notice the changes don't recognize them as symptoms of disease.

Acromegalics being treated at Grady Memorial Hospital in Atlanta are sometimes asked to come in on conference days to be seen by medical students from Morehouse School of Medicine and Emory University School of Medicine. For how can these students one day recognize an acromegalic if they have never seen one? A few men come and exhibit their bony faces to the curious students, but they are uneasy. "One guy always held a cigar in front of his jaw," says Dr. Ward, "It was never lit." Even in a medical setting, they protect themselves from stares. Women acromegalics typically don't come on conference days. The scrutiny of others is too painful for them.

The pain of acromegaly is reflected in our folk literature.

The fairy tale giant of fee-fie-foe-fum fame, we can reasonably suppose, had grown excessively tall but well-proportioned during his childhood. Without treatment for excess growth hormone, however, the disease had turned into acromegaly after the giant's growth plates had closed. He then developed enlarged lips and tongue, a jutting lower jaw, space between his teeth, a bulging forehead, and a frightening size. He was then not only tall but monstrous looking. No wonder he retreated to the top of a beanstalk where his behavior became increasingly anti-social.

One modern giant, apparently acromegalic, has dealt with his frightful proportions in another way. In his youth, he reached an unusual height, towering over his friends. Then, when his growth plates sealed, his bones grew much larger around, his facial features grew more prominent, and other organs were distended. The giant turned these distortions into entertainment assets. His enormous torso scantily covered, he stomps into a wrestling ring, snapping his oversized jaw at the television camera. He threatens his opponent with enormous spade-like hands, then seizes him and throws him into the air. As a professional wrestler, the acromegalic giant is making the most of what he's got.

Acromegalic History

The faces of acromegalics are seen in paintings and sculpture throughout history. A thirteenth-century figure on a flying buttress of the cathedral at Reims, France, for example, shows a woman with abnormally large shoulders and hip bones and an acromegalic face. She is holding her hand to her head as if she had an Excedrin headache, a common symptom of acromegaly because a pituitary tumor often causes painful pressure on adjacent tissue. (Noted and photographed in the early twentieth century, the acromegalic figure was gone from the cathedral after World War I.)

French neurologist Pierre Marie (1853-1940) was such an important early investigator of acromegaly that his colleagues tried to name the disease for him. About the same time, another disease he had investigated was being called Marie's Disease so a new name had to be chosen for the adult form of gigantism. In

1886 Marie described in accurate medical detail two women acromegalics aged 37 and 54. Photos of these women show faces very like the illustrations of witches in children's books. Each has a large nose, a fleshy scowl, and a jutting chin just crying out for a wart on the end. The bowed back which makes a witch seem especially threatening is typical of acromegalics. It is easy to imagine how such unfortunate women were feared by small children and misunderstood by all. Just as male giants and acromegalics played the heavies in folklore, so female acromegalics were cast in the roles of witches in fairy tales, offering poison apples to Snow White and locking up Hansel and Gretel.

In 1891, Marie's original account, augmented by additional cases and reassessments of patients in the literature, was published as a major work on acromegaly by Marie and his Brazilian pupil and collaborator, Jose Souza-Leite. In these descriptions it was noted that the sella turcica was enlarged in all dimensions and the size of the pituitary was as big as a pigeon's egg or even an apple. Intense thirst and copious urine, symptoms of diabetes, were also noted in many cases as well as "a want of sexual power." Marie proved the connection between acromegaly and a pituitary tumor but did not discover that the tumors caused hormone overproduction.

Another important work on acromegaly was the autobiography of Leonard Mark, M.D. (1855-1930). A physician at St. Bartholomew Hospital in London, Mark authored *Acromegaly, A Personal Experience*. He was probably first affected by the disease at about age 24 but did not recognize it until he was 50 when skeletal changes were obvious. He detailed the progression of his own acromegaly and obtained an X-ray showing his enlarged sella turcica. The autopsy, which he himself had ordered before his death, confirmed many other abnormalities which were the result of his disease.

By the end of the nineteenth century it was agreed that the pituitary was the growth center and that acromegaly was gigantism in adulthood.

Where Excess GH Comes From

Excess GH comes from an over-active pituitary gland. Very mild acromegaly, for example, sometimes occurs in pregnancy, when the pituitary is normally slightly enlarged, and subsides when the pregnancy is over. Most often excess levels of GH are caused by a benign pituitary tumor, also called an *adenoma*.

Tumors located in the anterior pituitary account for about 10% of all tumors located inside the skull. The abnormal growth may be derived from any of the five cell types which secrete hormones: lactotrophs, somatotrophs, thyrotrophs, gonadotrophs, and corticotrophs. The tumor more often than not begins to manufacture the same hormone as the healthy tissue from which it is derived. As the tumor grows, it can produce quantities far beyond normal.

Tumors of the lactotrophs or prolactin-secreting cells are the most common, accounting for 30% of all tumors in the anterior pituitary. Somatotrophs or GH-secreting cells are second, accounting for 20%; mixed prolactin and GH-secreting tumors account for 7%. Taken together, one out of four anterior pituitary tumors causes excess GH and acromegaly.

Rarely, a tumor of the lung or of the pancreatic islands produce GHRH (growth hormone releasing hormone), which, added to the GHRH normally released by the hypothalamus, stimulates the somatotrophs to oversecrete. Even more rarely, excessive GH production can be caused by a tumor derived from cells that do not usually produce GH. Thirty-five percent of tumors in the anterior pituitary are non-functional, that is, they manufacture no hormone at all. Causing no hormone-related symptoms, these are left untreated until they press against adjacent structures. When a tumor presses the pituitary too much, the result could be destruction and hypoactivity of the gland instead of hyperactivity.

How You Know For Sure

Most diagnosis of acromegaly is done by appearances. Older texts describe elaborate methods of testing for abnormal size, for example, dipping the hand of the patient into water and measuring the displacement of water or pinching flesh with calipers. But who knows how much water a patient's hand displaced before or how many centimeters of scowling brow is normal for him? Far more diagnostic are the before-and-after sizes of hats, rings, gloves, and shoes.

If appearances are not enough, it is easy to confirm or rule out acromegaly by a glucose suppression test. The patient takes 50 to 100 grams of glucose (sugar) in water by mouth and an hour later a sample of blood is drawn. After glucose loading, GH in healthy people should be less than 5 ng/ml (nanograms per milliliter). Values over 5 ng/ml suggest acromegaly. In borderline cases, thyrotropin releasing hormone (TRH) may be given to the patient; healthy people show no rise in GH after TRH while acromegalics show a marked rise.

In addition, an X-ray will show a distended sella turcica; a CT scan (cerebral computed tomography) will show tumors spilling out of the sella, and polytomography detects the tumor growing down through the sella floor into the nasal sinus. The possibility of a

GHRH-producing tumor of the pancreas should also be ruled out before invasive treatment of the pituitary.

What Can Be Done

The goals of treatment are to control tumor growth and to reduce the secretion of GH to normal levels. Transphenoidal (i.e., through the nose) microsurgery is the treatment of choice.

Originally, pituitary surgery was performed by opening the top of the skull. By the early twentieth century, a surgical approach through the mouth or nose made surgery more precise but the patient was not infrequently left with hypopituitary function. Today microsurgery through the nose is very effective and safe with few side effects. In most instances, pituitary function is not impaired.

Sometimes, however, surgery is not possible or fails to remove the entire tumor. Then other treatments are necessary. X-ray treatment has been used to slow tumor growth and hormone production, but pituitary adenomas are often resistant to radiation. Also, X-rays used with a heavy hand destroy normal pituitary function, leaving the patient deficient in all the trophic hormones and dependent on replacement therapy. Moreover, the benefits of radiation treatment are very slow in appearing. So X-ray treatment is rarely used and only where a center may have particular expertise with a proton-beam.

Bromocriptine is a dopamine-like drug that, used alone, lowers GH to normal levels in about 25% of acromegalic patients. This pharmaceutical approach may not reduce the size of the tumor so it is used after surgery or radiation for those who still have 10 ng/ml or more GH. Bromocriptine also reduces excess secretion of prolactin, the milk-producing hormone, which may accompany acromegaly.

The GH inhibiting factor, somatostatin, is a natural for reducing GH levels, but has a half-life of only three or four minutes. Octreotide, also called sandostatin, is a new synthetic variation of somatostatin that is sometimes effective in treating acromegaly when injected three times a day. Octreotide and bromocriptine together are sometimes the best pharmaceutical solution.

Surgical treatment brings immediate relief; other methods cause gradual improvement. Swelling of soft tissues resolve, headaches diminish, visual disturbance improves or disappears, excess sweating stops, and diabetes is cured. Patients report a new sense of well-being.

What Acromegaly Shows Us

The lesson of acromegaly to be heeded by all those who are considering growth hormone therapy, whether for short kids or for the elderly: Too much GH may be worse than no GH at all.

CHAPTER SIX

Tom Thumb and
Other Short Stories

Now some time after this, she had a little boy who was strong and healthy, but was no bigger than a thumb... They let him want for nothing, yet still the child grew no bigger, but remained the same size as when he was born. Still, he looked out on the world with intelligent eyes, and soon showed himself a clever and agile creature, who was lucky in all he attempted.

—Grimm's tale of Tom Thumb

There sat the unfortunate miller's daughter... She had not the least idea how to spin straw into gold, and she became more and more distressed, until at last she began to weep. Then all at once the door sprang open, and in stepped a little manikin (dwarf), who said: "Good evening, Mistress Miller, what are you weeping so for?"

—Grimm's tale of Rumpelstiltskin

Then she saw a little cottage and went into it to rest herself. Everything in the cottage was small, but neater and cleaner than can be told. There was a table on which was a white cover, and seven little plates, and on each plate a little spoon; moreover, there were seven little knives and forks, and seven little mugs. Against the wall stood seven

little beds side by side, and covered with snow-white
counterpanes... When it was quite dark the owners of the
cottage came back; they were seven dwarfs who dug and
delved in the mountains for ore.

—*Grimm's tale of Snow White*

From the malevolent Rumpelstiltskin to the cuddly
Seven Dwarfs, little people have starred in fairy
tales just as often as their giant counterparts. In Scandi-
navian and Teutonic folklore, tribes of dwarfs inhab-
ited the mountains and worked the mines. Dwarfs have
captured our imagination in different kinds of fiction.
Who can forget the little people who tied up the intrud-
ing Gulliver and whose house fire Gulliver put out
with the most convenient fire extinguisher? Who
doesn't remember the Teeny Weenies, those ingenious
little characters in the funny papers of our youth who
arranged air travel on robins' backs and drank from
acorn cups? While these last two tribes were impossi-
bly tiny and entirely fictional, some of the small characters of the fairy tales were based on the intriguing
and true existence of dwarfs.

Real life dwarfs have fascinated people of ordinary
size throughout the ages. Dwarfs played the role of
jesters in ancient China. Pictures in ancient Egyptian
tomb paintings and sculpture show "household
dwarfs" kept like pets. Less favored among the He-
brews, dwarfs, similar to others with "a blemish," were
not allowed to go into the temple and offer bread to
God. (Leviticus, XXI: 17, 20, and 23) However, Medvei
points out in *A History of Endocrinology* that Jesus favored Zacchaeus the publican who "was little of stat-

ure" and had climbed a sycamore tree to see Jesus over the crowd. Jesus said to Zacchaeus, "Make haste and come down; for today I must abide at thy house." It is not unlikely that Zacchaeus had chosen the despised profession of tax collector because he was already shunned for his small stature and might do no better.

The Romans of the same period, says Medvei, "were keen on cretinous dwarfs" and kept them around for entertainment. Slave children, it has been reported, were sometimes deliberately stunted to meet the demand for dwarfs. Household dwarfs were in vogue in Europe throughout the Renaissance as depicted in family scenes in paintings of the period. During the eighteenth and nineteenth centuries Russian czars and the nobility kept dwarfs and delighted particularly in dwarf weddings. Over the centuries only a few dwarfs were accepted as respected members of their communities; the rest were entertainers when lucky, outcasts when not in vogue.

In modern times, dwarfs still earn a living as entertainers, traveling with the great circuses and small roadside carnivals, and playing roles in television shows. However, an increasing acceptance of physical differences has allowed dwarfs to enjoy relatively normal lives in which dwarfism is only incidental.

Of all the kinds of dwarfs, the smallest are generally those perfectly proportioned dwarfs that lack growth hormone (GH).

According to Guinness...

The shortest mature human verified by independent sources was Pauline Musters. She was only 11.8 inches when she was born in 1876, according to Guinness. By age nine, she had reached 21.65 inches tall, about the length of a large newborn baby. The tiny Dutch woman died at age nineteen at 23.2 inches. At her top weight of nine pounds, she was somewhat overweight for her height, but still basically proportionate.

The shortest adult male dwarf was Calvin Phillips of Bridgewater, Massachusetts. He weighed only two pounds at birth in 1791 and stopped growing at age five at 26 1/2 inches.

The smallest living dwarf is Nelson de la Rosa (born in 1968), who stands only 28.3 inches tall as measured by the director of the medical association in his native country, Santo Domingo. The perfectly proportioned young man, weighing 15 pounds, can easily get a lift from his normal-sized siblings.

Unlike giants, who tend to die young, many dwarfs have a normal life expectancy. At least two female dwarfs have made it to age 100.

The dwarf with the most unusual history was Adam Rainer who at age twenty-one measured just under 3 feet 11 inches. But then his growth hormone status reversed itself and he took off growing. By age thirty-two, he was 7 feet 1 3/4 inches and when he died at age fifty-one, he was 7 feet 8 inches. Rainer, according to Guinness, was thus the only person to be both a dwarf and a giant.

The Real Tom Thumb

The most famous dwarf was undoubtedly Tom Thumb, nicknamed for the little guy in the fairy tale. He was born Charles Stratton in 1838. Helen Reeder Cross in her book *The Real Tom Thumb*, gives us a glimpse of his childhood:

Charles struggled to get out of the doll bed. Every time he got a good grip on the side of the cradle, his sister pushed him in the stomach till he collapsed in angry cries. "I don't want to be the baby," he screamed, tearing a baby bonnet off his head. "But you have to be the baby," she insisted. Their mother came to Charles's rescue, picking up her four-year-old son and setting him in a miniature chair pushed up to a miniature table and pushed some books in front of him. "Here, read these," she said.

Charles at four years of age was very bright, but he had not grown an inch since he was five months old. His sister's forcing him to play the baby in her childish games was the least of injuries to his dignity. The neighbors in their small town of Stockbridge, Connecticut, whispered about him as he passed, and children taunted him.

That year the famed showman Phinneas T. Barnum, hearing of Charles' 24-inch stature, came to see if the carpenter's son was right for his American Museum in New York. Although at first skeptical, thinking Charles might have a sudden growth spurt, Barnum was won over by Charles' personality and presence. Given the stage name of General Tom Thumb, the talented dwarf set out to win hearts with his song, dance, and comedy act. Then he traveled to all the world capitals. He charmed Queen Victoria and all of London, conquered France, then watched a bullfight from the Spanish Queen Isabella's lap. Back in the United States, Barnum took Tom and the rest of his museum show on the road, the first large American circus. While in Washington, Tom met President Abraham Lincoln, who is said to have remarked to his small visitor, "You and I are the long and the short of it, I guess."

In 1863 Tom Thumb married a lady, who measured 2 feet 8 inches, in what appears to have been a true love match. He and his tiny bride, Lavinia, greeted guests to their wedding reception standing on a grand piano.

The world's most famous midget and his wife wanted to look their friends in the eye.

Though talented and attractive, rich and beloved, Tom, at the height of success, nevertheless lamented to his mentor, Barnum, that he was lonely because his size—he eventually reached 3 feet 4 inches—cut him off from normal satisfactions. "I cannot even ask you, my oldest and best friend, to eat with me at my own table," he said, noting that Barnum could not have fit in his scaled down home or its miniature table and chairs.

In contrast to Cross's account, the *Guinness Book of World Records* gives a harsher edge to Tom's friendship with his mentor Barnum: "...he came into the clutches of the circus proprietor P.T. Barnum," says Guinness of Barnum's relationship with the small performer.

Whether Tom's circus career represented opportunity or exploitation, few abnormally small people can take their predicament on the road as successfully as Tom Thumb did. However, in recent years, several well known entertainment personalities have done extremely well because of or in spite of dwarfism. Child-star Gary Coleman, whose growth was interrupted by kidney disease, seemed precocious on stage and screen because of his small stature. The cute little-kid image of the star of the television comedy series "Different Strokes" waned only when his voice changed and his size was more readily recognized as a disorder.

Grandeur at an Early Age

The story of another very small person, the talented character actress Linda Hunt, lends insight into the experience of being abnormally small. A friend of Hunt's confided this to Cynthia Zarin, the author of a profile of Hunt in *The New Yorker*: "Think of it—the premium that is placed on personal appearance for actors. Instead of deciding to become something where personal appearance wouldn't mean anything, (Hunt) said, 'People are staring at me. I am going to make that my profession and turn it into an art.' It's an extraordinary decision. It's an outrageously defiant decision."

The diminutive Hunt has had big roles written specifically for her. Arthur Miller wrote the starring role of a female jockey in the television play "Fame" for Hunt, and George Trow wrote "The Tennis Game" for her to play the lead. She has been equally successful in wildly diverse plays and movies in which her small stature, 4 feet 9 inches, adds an interesting dimension—for example, in the role of Queen Elizabeth I in "Elizabeth Dead" and of Nurse Hooper in the movie "She-Devil."

Hunt won an Academy Award for her performance as the oriental dwarf photographer, Billy Kwan, in Peter Weir's 1982 movie, "The Year of Living Dangerously." Weir cast her after rejecting dozens of small male actors. He had been negative at first about casting a woman, but Hunt soon won him over by her understanding of the dwarf's character.

As a baby in 1945 Linda Hunt had seemed slow to develop and was taken to a doctor at age six months. The doctor made the diagnosis of *cretinism*, a disease of insufficient thyroid hormone during pregnancy and early life, and he offered this baby no hope of normal height or intelligence. He was wrong about everything but the height, of course. Her small size was correctly attributed to low GH production only when Hunt was in her early teens, about the same time Raben first used GH experimentally with a GH-deficient child. The hormone was not available outside of research.

By the time Hunt turned sixteen, however, human pituitary GH was being used, when available, to make such children grow, and Hunt belatedly got intensive treatment. The treatments did little good although her growth plates evidently remained open as in a younger child. Hunt recalls for the *New Yorker* profile how she and a close friend plotted a trick on the staff during one of her stays in the hospital where her GH-treatment was being monitored. "We cooked up this idea that Dana would sleep in my bed, and the nurses would see her when they came in in the morning. Dana is almost six feet tall, and big all over, and she has strawberry-blond hair. 'It's worked!' they would say."

But Hunt soon tired of the useless medical interventions.

"When I was twenty-five, I put my foot down and said *no*. My sense of it was that I just wanted to be left alone to find out who I was."

Hunt is described, says Zarin, as "full of secret energy." Others say she has "dignity and stillness" and an "air of being on top of things," pun perhaps intended. Others speak of her "authority." Authority, explains Hunt, is "what I developed to survive. To survive what I was—how I was different from everyone else. I had this perception in the air around me that there was something wrong with me, and I knew that what was wrong with me *wasn't* wrong with anyone else. And I saw that if you talk in a loud voice people will think you have something to say, so I cultivated a loud voice. And I learned to say all my vowels and consonants. I developed grandeur at a very early age. Say, four. I saw my parents as safe and secure, too. But I knew that for me it wasn't going to be enough to be a grownup. I was going to have to be a duchess."

Most dwarfs are neither duchess nor actor. One might be your dry cleaner or dentist or next door neighbor. Unlike giants, dwarfs are generally normal in achievement and socialization.

CHAPTER SIX

Dwarfs, Midgets, and Just Little People

One dwarf, a successful entrepreneur in Chapel Hill, North Carolina, had been a popular cheerleader while a student at the University of North Carolina and was later elected to the legislature of that state. Then he became the owner of a hobby supply store. He would sit on a high stool by the cash register. First-time customers asked him where to find a particular item and he offered to locate it for them. To the customers' astonishment, when he jumped down off the stool, he completely disappeared from view behind the counter. They waited in puzzlement not knowing where he had gone. Only when he emerged around the end of the counter did they realize he was a dwarf. His small size no doubt challenged him but has certainly not inhibited him from considerable success.

Such dwarfs, often about the size of an average kindergarten child, have defective cartilage cells at the ends of some of their bones so that these cells do not multiply no matter how much GH they may have had in their blood. Their children may also be dwarfs. The genetic limitation in the ability of certain cartilage cells to respond to normal growth signals is called *achondroplasia* or *hypochondroplasia* and results in a normal or large size head and disproportionately short long bones. The Seven Dwarfs of Snow White fame probably represent achondroplastic or hypochondroplastic dwarfs also, judging by the way they rocked from side to side when they walked—at least in the Disney version—and their probable blood relationship.

There are perhaps a half million dwarfs of all types in the United States. About 5,000 belong to Little People of America, a national organization with regional and local chapters that offers fellowship, support, and

113

information to members, all people under 4 feet 10 inches. The term "little people" is the expression preferred, according to one source, by most undersized people in the world. However, Little People of America uses the word *dwarf* in some of its literature including a book entitled me *My Child Is a Dwarf*. The word *midget* has been used to mean proportionate dwarf (for example, the GH-deficient) while *dwarf* has meant either all little people or disproportionate little people.

Only a few of those who experience dwarfism suffer from a deficiency in growth hormone. Other causes include other hormonal disorders, for instance, too little thyroxine in cretinism or too much cortisol in Cushing's Disease. Malnutrition, deprived environment, or serious disease may cause a failure to grow. Sometimes a gene deletion on an individual's chromosomes, the building blocks of heredity, eliminates the possibility of normal growth.

When a genetic "defect," because of inbreeding, becomes the norm for a group of people who function successfully, this group can be considered a separate race. Races of very small people in Asia and Africa were described in the first century A.D. by Pliny, prolific Roman natural historian and naval commander. The average male height of both Asian and African pygmies is four and a half feet with many much smaller. Both groups have dark skin and similar facial characteristics. Although being generally proportionate, they have unusually long arms and large feet with long, supple toes which they use skillfully in climbing trees. The pygmy groups in Asia are called Negritos and are biologically unrelated to the pygmies of the African jungles.

It had been suggested that pygmies are inbred tribes with genetically transmitted growth hormone deficiency. Recent studies, however, show that African pygmies have normal or even high levels of GH in their blood. Experimental treatment of young African pygmies with GH had no effect on their growth, which suggests an inherited defect in GH receptors. But small stature can hardly be considered a defect when these tiny people thrive in the jungle where larger Africans fear to go. Lithe, quick, and strong, they bring down large game with tiny poisoned arrows and even kill huge elephants.

Small size without disability is an issue only where the rest of society is larger and tall stature is prized.

Kids, Growth, and GH

Every child is a potential dwarf. To grow into a full-sized adult, a child must have sufficient nourishment, good health, genetic integrity, time—and growth hormone. A child lacking any one or more of these necessities will experience limited skeletal growth.

Children with growth hormone (GH) deficiency represent only a small percentage of short children. One out of ten children who fall below the first percentile in height is GH-deficient, and one out of fifty children who fall below the fifth percentile is GH-deficient. GH-deficiency is an important cause of small stature because its effects can be extreme.

Failure to grow at a normal rate may be the only sign of isolated GH-deficiency. GH-deficient children typically grow less than 4 cm (1.6 inches) per year. When the depressed growth rate is noted and when the child's height begins to fall from its initial channel into lower height percentiles, GH-deficiency may be suspected. An infantile appearance sometimes described as "cherub-like" because of small facial bones and an abnormal retention of body fat are also clues to GH-deficiency.

GH-deficient children typically have a significantly

delayed bone age. Bone age reflects the degree to which the cartilage at the ends of bones has hardened causing the epiphyses or growth plates to approach closure. Bone age is determined largely by the combined action of sex steroids, thyroid hormones, and GH. Ultimate height is determined by the combination of growth velocity and bone age maturation. Normally, bone age matches chronological age. In treating GH-deficient children, doctors must pay attention not only to growth but how fast the bone age is advancing. Therapy is best begun at an early bone age and may continue until the epiphyses close, whatever age that may be.

"Typical" GH-Deficient Child Is an Individual.

Michael's parents did not suspect their second son had a growth problem until he was eight years old because the whole family is small—mother Wendy is 5 feet 2, his father is 5 feet 6 1 1/2 inches, and his older brother is in the lower percentiles of height as expected. Besides, an earlier illness seemed to account for some delay in Michael's growth. Wendy's first hint of a growth disorder came, she says, when, "like a good Jewish mother, I bought Michael's school clothes at end-of-the-year sales one size larger than what he was wearing. I expected him to grow into them by the time school started the next year." But the year Michael was eight years old, wearing a size 6, he never grew into those new clothes. She took him to her pediatrician who confirmed that Michael had grown only a half inch in a year. His height had fallen from the neatly marked lower channels of the growth chart into the bottomless space below.

A pediatric endocrinologist to whom Michael was referred confirmed that the slow growth was abnormal, noting that Michael's bone age was three years behind his chronological age. When tests proved Michael was a GH-deficient child, he prescribed GH injections. Michael cried for two hours before the appointment for his first injecton. No, he didn't like being called "shrimp" at school, but for the moment he liked the idea of shots even less. Wendy wasn't crazy about giving Michael his first injection herself, but with the doctor guiding the syringe and giving her encouragement, she managed. Michael's father watched a video of the procedure seven times before he dared do it himself. At age eleven, during a visit to his doctor's office, Michael first saw the Inject-Ease (R), a device from Palco Laboratories that automatically, quickly, and relatively painlessly penetrates the skin when a little button is pressed. Once he experienced the Inject-Ease, Michael decided he was ready to give himself the shots.

"Michael likes to be in control of his world, and giving himself the shots makes him feel in control," says Wendy, who usually draws the GH into the needle for him. "He even has his special way of doing it."

Michael swabs the spot he will inject with alcohol and then draws a ring around the spot with a marker so he won't lose the place while the alcohol dries. Then he positions the device carefully, pushes the button that releases the needle, barely wincing, and finally pushes the plunger. Then he takes the swab, still moist with alcohol, and erases the colored circle. It's a ritual that gives him some satisfaction.

Even so, the regime is not easy, and when the doctor recommended Michael increase shots from six days a week to every day, he balked. He treasured that Sunday off. A compromise was reached, and Michael now gets one day a month off.

The diligence has paid off. In the first two years of

GH therapy Michael grew seven inches. After three years Michael is just a hair under the 5th percentile line that once seemed so distant. After his first day of tennis classes last summer, he announced at home that it was the first time he had joined a new group that no one had exclaimed, "But you are too little to be eleven!"

Michael's doctor plans to keep him on GH until he reaches bone age 16. Hand X-rays show Michael's bone age is still almost 3 years behind. With this prolonged treatment, his doctor expects Michael to reach his genetic potential, an ultimate height of 5 feet 8, a little taller than his dad.

Diagnosis in Infancy: the Cutting Edge

A child born growth hormone deficient is not usually small at birth, however, because other factors than GH, mostly maternal factors like nutrition and the efficiency of the placenta, are more important to growth before and shortly after birth. Placental GH is quite high in the mother's blood during the last weeks of pregnancy while her pituitary GH is undetectable. Thirty minutes after delivery of the baby, placental GH disappears from the mother's blood, its source swept out with the baby. Moreover, whatever the prenatal GH status before birth, hypothalamic/pituitary damage may be done during birth. The most common cause of GH-deficiency in infancy, in fact, is an interruption of the oxygen supply or trauma during the birth process. Other causes are genetic or disease related. In any case, events that damage the potential for GH production do not necessarily make the babies smaller at birth. Some pituitary dwarfs have started out as whopping nine-pounders. These are rarely diagnosed in infancy because who would think such a big baby—or any average sized baby—has a growth problem.

But occasionally a very young infant deficient in GH has been diagnosed and treated. The second son of a Dutch family—let's call him Franz—was lucky enough to begin GH treatment when he was only nine weeks old—just beginning to smile—thanks to an international team of doctors. Now thriving, Franz is expected to reach his genetic potential in height. This infant received treatment so early because of the lessons doctors learned from his older brother—we'll call him Hans.

Hans was born a normal-sized baby but soon stopped growing. When Hans was three, he was the size of an average nine-month-old baby. Of course, his family and doctors knew something was wrong. Tests showed he was deficient in thyroid hormones and this at first seemed to account for his growth retardation. Treatment with thyroxin corrected some of Hans' health problems, but still he did not grow. Then the pediatric endocrinologist, J.M. Wit of Utrecht, realized that Hans' pituitary gland was not making significant amounts of growth hormone either. Hans was said to have multi-pituitary deficiency which means he lacked more than one pituitary hormone. Dr. Wit put Hans on GH therapy and the little fellow began to grow. Unfortunately, Hans is still quite short because he experienced puberty at a normal age, his growth plates closed, and further treatment could not make him grow any taller.

But when little Franz was born, Dr. Wit was ready for him. Not only had Dr. Wit treated Franz's older brother, but he had treated another family with two children both deficient in pituitary hormones. He realized that the disorder could be genetic. When Franz was born and gave signs of being hypoglycemic, Dr. Wit gave him a full battery of the latest tests, which enabled the

Dutch pediatric endocrinologist to verify that he, too, was growth hormone-deficient before any growth deficit could be detectable.

Dr. Wit also consulted with Dr. John Parks, researcher in pediatric endocrinology at Emory University School of Medicine, who teamed up with Dr. Roland Pfaffle, a German researcher in the same field. In 1991, Pfaffle succeeded in identifying the exact gene defect that caused the GH-deficiency in these boys and in the children of the other family. "The same DNA techniques that enable synthesis of human GH can be used in research to understand what's wrong in genetic forms of GH deficiency," says Parks. While the team is proud to have intervened so soon after Franz' birth, Parks predicts that some day, because of this work, physicians will be able to diagnose this genetic growth defect while the baby is still in the womb.

Normal or Deficient?
It's Not Black and White.

As long as there has been GH therapy, parents of very short children have wanted the treatment for their children. And as long as there has been GH therapy, treatment has been limited by FDA guidelines to children like Michael, Hans, and Franz—children with clear GH deficiency.

Before 1963 the diagnosis of GH deficiency was based on height, appearance, and medical history; these are still of paramount importance. When tests became available to aid in diagnosis, GH deficiency was defined as no measurable GH production, not only because the tests were not sensitive enough to distinguish low levels of GH production, but because of the scarcity of the hormone. The supply was to be saved for the most clearly GH-deficient. Certainly there were doctors who administered GH to those outside the guidelines but for the most part the key to therapy was a positive diagnosis of GH-deficiency by testing.

Testing, Testing

Today, even with unlimited amounts of GH available, the only indication for GH therapy approved by the FDA and the majority of physicians is still a positive diagnosis of GH-deficiency (or inadequacy, as the FDA calls it) verified by testing. GH therapy is generally replacement therapy. To give GH therapy to non-deficient patients is perhaps to risk the dangers of acromegaly; cardiovascular damage, enlarged heart, and insulin-resistance. Therefore, at present, to become a candidate for GH-therapy, a child must test GH-deficient.

There are two basic kinds of tests for GH-deficiency. One type is *spontaneous* testing of GH production and the other is *stimulation* testing of GH production.

In spontaneous tests, blood is drawn from the patient in several samples, for example, every twenty minutes for four hours during the day or as a 12-hour overnight sampling study. Spontaneous tests can also last 24 hours. Basing a decision on a spontaneous test is difficult, however, because of the natural ebb and flow in GH secretion. If a sample is taken during a normal dip in the GH secretory pattern and no GH is found, can you call a patient GH-deficient? Of course not. In fact, says Susan Rose, M.D. (then at the National Institutes of Health, now at the University of New Mexico), "Attempts to use measurements of growth hormone in samples obtained at random times or at timed intervals after the onset of sleep have failed because the pulsatile nature of growth hormone secretion produced an unacceptably high incidence of false positive results" for GH-deficiency.

Stimulation tests seem to solve some of the problems spontaneous tests do not address. Ideally you test for GH when GH is at its highest level. With stimulation tests, instead of guessing at that peak time, you provoke it. In a stimulation test, the patient is given a substance or activity that is known to stimulate a substantial GH response.

Over the years an interesting succession of stimulation methods have been tried with varying success. A beef broth was developed in England that, when consumed, brought on a surge of GH in 93% of the children tested, making it one of the safest and most effective stimulants. The broth was abandoned because many of the children refused to drink the less than tasty stock. Another stimulant, the simplest and most natural of all, is exercise: One investigator found riding bikes "as far as the children could reasonably tolerate" resulted in 91% of his young subjects reaching a satisfactory GH surge, while another researcher got his patients to run up and down three flights of hospital stairs four times to achieve GH elevations. This worked as a screening device—those patients who experienced a surge of GH were not deficient—and recently there has been renewed interest in standardizing exercise tests.

In standard practice, injection of various substances known to stimulate GH will define GH-deficiency. One of these substances is arginine, the protein in the drink the vendors offered on the Capitol Mall to stimulate GH. Other substances administered intravenously to induce a burst of GH are levodopa (L.dopa), clonidine, ornithine, glucagon, and insulin.

After stimulation by any one of these substances, 75% to 90% of normal children will show a rise in GH.

Any two tests will provoke at least one adequate GH response in virtually all patients with normal GH. A diagnosis of GH-deficiency is made when kids fail to secrete GH at an appropriate level, generally defined as between 8 and 10 ng/ml, on two successive tests using different sources of stimulation.

"Multiple stimuli induce GH release, but insulin-induced hypoglycemia usually is considered the 'gold standard,'" say E.O. Reiter and P.M. Martha of Tufts University in a 1990 review. Pediatric endocrinologist Stephen Anderson uses the insulin-induced hypoglycemia test coupled with the L. dopa test to determine GH deficiency. This is how it works:

Six-year-old Frances has come to Dr. Anderson's office for these tests. For comfort, she has brought along her big brown teddy bear, Bo. When she and Bo settle into the blue leather recliner for the test, it is difficult to tell who is the patient. The two of them begin to watch video cartoons while a nurse administers the first test. In the insulin-induced hypoglycemia test, symptomatic low blood sugar is induced in the patient by an injection of insulin. Within a half hour of the injection, the patient becomes very uncomfortable—restless, shaky, and sweating. If Frances's pituitary responds properly, this biochemical stress will cause her pituitary to secrete GH and also adrenocorticotropic hormone (ACTH) at peak levels. When this secretory reaction kicks in, after about ten minutes, she will feel more comfortable. The surge of GH and of cortisol from the adrenal glands define normal pituitary secretion. But Frances does not secrete GH normally and the GH peaks never occur. If she also fails to produce GH during the L. dopa test which follows, Dr. Anderson will conclude that she does not have the capability of producing GH. The insulin glucose test is potentially dangerous for those with ACTH deficiency as well as uncomfortable and Dr. Anderson keeps a syringe of injectable glucose (sugar) handy in case the patient becomes seriously hypoglycemic (low on blood sugar), but he has only had to use it once in ten years. Frances does just fine. She sniffles and clings more tightly to Bo the bear as the discomfort subsides.

Stimulation vs Spontaneous

In 1984 a subset of children were discovered who passed the stimulation tests, but whose growth had stopped and in addition were known to have suffered damage to the hypothalamic/pituitary axis. These children were leukemia patients who had been treated by cranial radiation. These children seemed to be GH deficient by their heights and low growth velocity. Yet they passed the stimulation tests. Those old tests of spontaneous secretion, however, showed that over a period of time the children simply were no longer releasing GH. This subset, said to have *neurosecretory dysfunction*, was considered GH-deficient, was treated with GH, and responded. Radiation treatment has become an increasingly common cause of GH-deficiency. Perhaps more important to the larger picture, the discovery of children who were otherwise provably GH-deficient but who tested negative on stimulation tests opened up the possiblilty that the stimulation tests may have been missing some other subsets of children.

In the meantime other confusing factors were becoming increasingly evident. When radioimmunoassays (RIA) for GH, the tests that actually detected GH in the sample, were first developed in the late 60s, they were fairly similar and produced comparable results from laboratory to laboratory and test time to test time. But as techniques proliferated, significantly variable results appeared among the different labs and even the different lab technicians.

Another confusing factor, experts of all persuasions admitted, was that no one really knew what was the "normal" level of GH production for a particular pre-pubertal child, let alone one in the unpredictable throes of puberty.

Doubt was also cast on the dividing line between GH-deficient and GH-sufficient, set in the era when the hormone was very scarce. Indeed, most doctors are stretching the old definition of GH-deficiency, which they think is no longer appropriate.

In the confusion, several groups have been lead to explore the possibility of finding new subsets of children who could be diagnosed GH-deficient and treated with GH. One of these groups with much to gain is the drug companies who would profit from broadening the market beyond patients for whom the drug was developed. Another group includes researchers whose careers hinge on finding new wrinkles, perhaps even new worlds to investigate through experimental medicine. A third group is made of parents of very short children who are hoping GH can help their child. A fourth group includes clinical physicians tired of saying, "Yes, your child is very, very short but there is nothing I can do."

Hoping to end the argument about spontaneous testing vs stimulation testing, at least, Rose et al. did a careful study of 54 short children, controlling the variables of puberty, chronological age, and bone age. She demonstrated that stimulation tests identified all the GH-deficient children that had been identified by spontaneous tests and some additional ones that the spontaneous tests had missed. She concluded that the decision to use GH treatment should continue to be based on stimulation tests. Still the literature, particularly European, is full of mention of those short children who do not test deficient on stimulation tests but who demonstrate deficiency on tests of spontaneous GH production.

Rose adds, however, "The superior diagnostic accuracy of growth-hormone-stimulation tests should not obscure several concerns that emphasize the need for further improvements in diagnosis. First, ...limits for normal responses to the stimulation tests have not been established as a function of age, sex, and pubertal stage in normally growing children. Thus, rigorous criteria for what constitutes an abnormal response have not yet been developed. Second, many stimulation tests are available. However, the relative diagnostic accuracy of the various tests and combinations of tests has not been systematically evaluated. Third, the performance of different radio-immunoassays of growth hormone varies, and this has hindered the development of uniform diagnostic criteria."

If They Grow...

Finally, in the uncertainty over testing, some experts in Europe, especially, but also a minority in the U.S. finally said in so many words: So much for GH tests. Let's just try short kids on GH and if they grow, they must need it.

After all, says M. Vanderschueren-Lodeweyckx of the University of Leuven, Belgium, "The value of GH secretion assessment is to show whether the patient will indeed benefit from treatment with hGH." With that opinion, the Belgian expert has stepped off the pier into the sea of controversy, as we shall see particularly in the next chapter.

Who Got the GH-Deficient Diagnosis?

In October 1985 when Protropin®, the biosynthetic hGH from American drug manufacturer Genentech, was approved by the FDA for clinical use, almost 6,000 short patients in the U.S. started the new GH-treatment together. For the next two years, in a survey by Gilbert August, M.D., et al., demographic data were taken from patients at 112 medical centers representing 40% of the total. The number of subjects was large enough to make even small differences between subsets significant.

Who were they, these kids who were recognized as abnormally short, were diagnosed as GH-deficient, and were seeking treatment? Were they the same as those who needed treatment? Or did their numbers reflect biases of doctors or parents?

Boys outnumbered girls more than two to one. Although some screening studies have shown that almost twice as many boys actually do suffer from GH-deficiency as girls, other findings of August et al. suggest some degree of bias based on gender. The girls with GH-deficiency of unknown origin were shorter for their sex when their problem was discovered than the boys were; apparently the girls experienced depressed growth longer before anyone noticed it and sought treatment.

A gender bias, if one exists, is no surprise. In our culture, it is more important for a boy to be reasonably tall than a girl. A short boy suffers socially more than a short girl and the likelihood of his becoming a leader is more diminished.

A difference in diagnosis by race was also explored. The patients who started GH treatment in the study years were 87.8% white, 6.0% black, 1.0% Asian, and

5.2% "other." Hispanic children were divided in unknown proportions between white and "other." At the
time, 12.9% of the U.S. population younger than 19
years old was black. Half as many blacks as should be
expected were in the treatment group. Black children,
like girls, were also significantly shorter at diagnosis of
GH-deficiency of unknown origin. Again, it is possible
that black children have less GH-deficiency than white
children, but it is more likely that black children were
not seeking diagnosis or getting treatment at the same
rate as white children.

Although ability to pay was not investigated in this
study, it is obvious that costs of diagnosis and treatment have been major factors keeping some who
needed GH treatment from getting it.

Goals

Before starting treatment, a child and his parents
may well wonder how they will define success. How
tall will the child have to be to be worth the sting of
hundreds of injections and the payment of thousands
of dollars a year for treatment? Is any increase in
growth worth the trouble?

J. M. Tanner, now professor emeritus of the Institute
of Child Health, University of London, and visiting
professor of auxology at the School of Public Health,
University of Texas, Houston, said in 1986 in an introduction to material provided doctors by Genentech:

> The prime objective of the treatment is to make the child
> grow to a final adult height which is the full height of the
> child's genetic potential. However, we are also interested
> in short term growth, to make a child's stature more nearly
> appropriate for his age at least for a time, even if this
> cannot be entirely sustained. The nearer a child's stature
> is to being appropriate for age, the better.

Although, in theory, reaching the child's genetic potential has always been the goal of GH therapy, in practice, prior to the availability of biosynthetic GH, two-thirds of children treated with pituitary GH wound up below the fifth percentile. In fact, treatment with pituitary GH often stopped when children reached a "normal" height of about the fifth percentile in order to make the hormone available for others more in need.

Today many GH-deficient children reach the goal of their genetic potential. Doctors and parents together, when considering treatment of a short child, make a determination of target height which under optimum circumstances is defined as the mid-parental average, the expected adult height based on a genetic contribution of both parents. A way of figuring the mid-parental average and putting it on a growth chart is offered by Parks in Chapter 10. Another way of figuring a range of projected adult height based on parental height is offered by J. M. Tanner.

First, figure the mid-parental average by adding together the heights of the child's mother and the child's father and divide the sum by two. For boys, the range of expected adult height or *parental target range* will be from 3.5 centimeters less than the mid-parental average to 16.5 cm. more than the mid-parental average. For girls the range will be from 15.5 cm. less than the mid-parental average to 2.5 cm. more. Final adult height for 95 per cent of normal children is expected to be within this range.

For example, John and Trish wonder how tall their children are expected to grow. Let's figure for them:

John's height is 5 feet 8 1/4 inches or   173.3 cm.
Trish's height is 5 feet 1 inch   or   + 154.9 cm.
                                             328.2 cm.

Divide the sum by 2 and you get 164.1 cm. or the mid-parental range.

Now figure the range in which John and Trish's son's height will most likely fall:

	164.1 cm.		164.1 cm.
	- 3.5 cm.		+16.5 cm.
Between	160.6 cm.	and	180.6 cm.
or between	5 ft. 3 in.	and	5 ft. 11 in.

Next figure the range in which John and Trish's daughter's height will most likely fall:

	164.1 cm.		164.1 cm.
	- 15.5 cm.		+ 2.5 cm.
Between	148.6 cm.	and	166.0 cm.
or between	4 ft. 10.5 in.	and	5 ft. 5.5 in.

Tanner suggests also that an appropriate amount be added to the projected height if the parents are believed not to have reached their own genetic height for whatever reason. Also, in this country and others, there is a trend for children to be a centimeter or two taller than their parents. This might be reason to raise the projected height a similar amount.

The Bottom Line: GH Therapy Works.

Kids taking GH grow, no doubt about it. Small clinical trials had, of course, proved treatment of GH-deficient children with biosynthetic GH was both effective and safe well before the FDA approval for nationwide clinical use. Still it was exciting to researchers when a great "freshman" class of 6,000 short kids in the U.S. started long term treatment with unlimited quantities of GH. Many of their counterparts in Europe were beginning the same route.

Comparing the Old and the New

The first question researchers and consumers asked was would the man-made hormone work as well as the natural stuff made in the human pituitary? The answer seemed to be, "Better."

Some patients, who had been treated with pituitary GH and stopped treatment when the natural hormone was banned, resumed treatment with biosynthetic GH. In one study in 1987, according to J. R. Bierich of the University of Tubingen, Germany, such children responded with an initial growth spurt of 10.7 cm (4.21 inches) per year which leveled off to 8.5 cm (3.35 inches) per year. But these GH therapy veterans were far outdone by the newcomers. When patients who had never received pituitary GH got the new stuff, they jumped to an initial rate of 14.9 cm (5.87 inches) per year which leveled off to a rate of 12 cm. (4.72 inches) per year. Both groups of short children were growing at a normal or above normal rate that put them well on their way to catching up to their normal agemates.

Can we conclude that the factory-made GH was even better than the natural product made by the human body?

"It is unlikely that any biosynthetic product should have a greater effect than the natural hGH," says Bierlich, concluding that the better results should be attributed to "the more physiological mode of administration."

The new mode of administration included differences in dose, frequency of administration, and method of injection. The oldest studies used the same fixed dose for all the children, while the new studies used a dose tailored to the child's weight. Even when GH began to be administered in weight-dependent doses, the relative dosages were half of what they are today. In older studies the recommended weekly weight-dependent dose of 1.5 mg/kg was divided up and administered three times during the week; in more recent studies, the weekly dose of 3.0 mg/kg was divided up and administered six times during the week. Moreover, clinical trials today are done with subcutaneous injection rather than with the more painful intramuscular injection favored in earlier years. Also, it should be noted that the new studies, on the average, started short children on GH treatment about a year younger than many previous studies.

The most recent studies leave comparisons with pituitary hormone behind in the realm of history and focus on finding the optimum parameters of treatment for each age.

Getting the Most Out of GH

The slowest growers get the biggest boost out of GH.

"We have shown that pretreatment height velocity is the major contributing factor to growth response..." says F. Darendeliler. He and his colleagues at Middlesex Hospital in London studied 90 prepubertal children divided into groups according to how fast they had been growing before treatment. He treated them all six times a week with a wide range of doses per unit of body weight. All the children responded to the GH treatment. Using a complex statistical analysis, he confirmed that the slowest growing group of children had the greatest growth response to treatment; the moderately growing children showed a moderate response;

and the fastest growing group showed the least growth response to treatment.

Dose

As recently as 1989 Darendeliler said, "In spite of the number of studies about growth hormone (GH) treatment, there is still uncertainty about the dose of GH required to promote growth... This is because the diagnostic criteria of the patients selected for GH treatment and their pretreatment auxological data [auxology is the science of measuring growth] differed widely; fixed dose regimens of GH used in several studies took into account neither the change in size of a developing child nor the observation that GH secretion increases with age and puberty...finally, the frequency of GH administration, which is known to exert an effect on growth response was not standardized. Not surprisingly, it has not been possible to demonstrate a consistent dose-response relationship for GH treatment."

Within each group, the dose of GH was the biggest factor in determining response. From this study Darendeliler produced a series of dose-response curves for differing pretreatment growth rates so that GH replacement can be better tailored to the individual.

Another researcher asked the question differently. If you give a particular child more GH will that child grow more? Yes, in the first year of treatment. After the first year of treatment, the dose and growth rate were not correlated. Even in the first year, the difference in growth rate is smaller than the change in dose. For example, in one study doubling the dose increased the growth rate only 1.6 times; a 3.3 fold increase in dose increased the growth rate only 2.3 times, and so forth. But doubling the dose does double the cost!

Frequency

Experimentation has consistently shown that the same amount of total weekly hormone (or even less) divided into more frequent injections is more effective than less frequent injections. Six or seven times a week or daily injections is now preferred over three times a week by most pediatric endocrinologists, even though FDA-approved labels on Protropin and Humatrope®, the GH product of Indianapolis drug manufacturer Eli Lilly, still say three times a week.

If daily injections were more effective than three times weekly, some researchers wondered if twice daily would be even better. Fortunately for the kids, studies showed twice-daily injections were no more effective than once daily injections. A regimen of daily doses given in the evening mimics the nocturnal secretion of GH in a normal person and is considered optimal.

Does GH Keep on Working?

Patients treated with GH typically show a spurt of growth the first three to sixth months when GH treatment starts. After this growth spurt, the growth rate levels off at a lower rate. Some researchers interpret the initial spurt as catch-up growth such as experienced by a child recovering from an illness or after receiving thyroxine for hypothyroidism; they consider the subsequent waning effect natural and not a sign of failure of therapy. Other researchers say the body rapidly adapts to the hormone by responding with less growth; these investigators want to focus research on preventing the waning effect. Sometimes a brief pause in treatment sets up another growth spurt when treatment resumes; intermittent treatment has therefore been tried with mixed results generally favoring continuous treatment.

Bone Age Advancement

Another critical factor is the comparison of gain in height and advancement of bone age. Fortunately, when growth is slow because of GH-deficiency, bone age is usually behind schedule also. When GH is given as treatment, growth speeds up and so usually does bone development. The trick is to get a substantial increase of growth without inducing bone maturation and closure of the growth plates before desired growth has been achieved. Advancement in bone age during GH treatment generally is not alarming. In group studies the average increase in height is greater than the advance in bone age; however, the results have been variable from patient to patient. Some patients, about one-third, experience greater skeletal maturity, especially those in their first year of treatment and again after six or seven years of treatment, and those who at the same time used steroids or a drug designed to prevent the waning effect. The relative gain in bone age versus growth and its implications for treatment must be evaluated on an individual basis.

Puberty

The years of puberty present a special challenge to pediatric endocrinologists. During puberty, normal kids spontaneously secrete 1.5 to 2 times the amount of GH as prepubertal children—the frequency of surges are the same but the amount of secretion is greater. GH responses to stimulation tests during puberty are also greater. It follows that the dosage in GH therapy should be increased accordingly. Researchers studied the matter and disagreed. The most accepted opinion, however, is that if a normal growth rate compared to bone age is not achieved in a patient by the time of puberty (spontaneous or induced with hormones), an increase in GH dose by 1.5 to 2 times may be necessary.

Delayed puberty may be favorable for getting maximum growth, but most doctors recommend that boys with gonadotropin deficiency (which often accompanies GH-deficiency) start taking low doses of testosterone at bone age 12-13 to induce puberty, and girls with gonadotropin deficiency start taking estrogen at bone age 12. With this therapy, children may experience a desirable pubertal growth spurt as well as the same physical changes as boys and girls of the same age.

What Else Happens with GH Treatment?

GH deficient children tend to be flabby if not outright obese and their fat tends to gather around the gut. GH-deficient children are often "apples" (as opposed to "pears" who carry their fat more on hips and thighs). The apple or *android* body type (sometimes called abdominal or male pattern) in adults is associated with greater risks of high blood pressure, diabetes, stroke, and certain heart disorders. GH administration tends to correct that tendency to go to pot, as Rudman's elderly men found out. GH not only favors building of muscle over fat, but it tends to favor fat on the hips and legs over abdominal fat. This can be observed by measuring the fat at different sites on children before and after GH treatment and also by looking at the cells under a microscope. GH treatment makes abdominal fat cells smaller, but leaves the hip/thigh fat cells the same. These effects of GH treatment are generally considered positive.

The best news about GH treatment for GH-deficient kids has been the rarity of undesirable side effects.

However, some rare side effects have occurred and these should be noted: Sometimes patients on GH develop hypothyroidism, so thyroid function should be tested regularly. If insufficiency develops, thyroid hormone replacement should be given. Investigators have also found a slightly increased incidence of slipped growth plates at the top of the thigh bone in children treated with GH. To put this into perspective, Stephen Anderson says he has seen in ten years of pediatric endocrinology practice only one slipped growth plate in a patient taking GH, and this patient, being overweight, was particularly at risk anyway. Some degree of insulin resistance is another possible side effect to be monitored, but no diabetes has been reported in patients treated with the recommended dosage of GH. An increased incidence of ovarian cysts has also been noted with girls on GH.

The most serious question to be raised about GH treatment concerns 18 cases of leukemia reported in patients 10 to 23 years of age who were or had been treated with GH. Though a small proportion of the thousands of children treated with GH, this number is calculated to be 1.5 times the normal rate. Jean-Claude Job, summarizing the situation, noted five cases of leukemia in a group of *untreated* GH-deficient young people. It is not known if the increased incidence of leukemia is related to GH treatment, GH-deficiency itself, or neither.

Job concludes, "No metabolic, visceral or immunological side-effects have been found during the very protracted studies done for the trial of different brands of synthetic GH in GH-deficient patients." Some day other problems may be attributed to long-term GH use, but after thirty years of successful GH use with GH-deficient kids, any problems discovered in the future are likely to be few and minor.

Barking Up a New Tree: The Role of GHRH

Another whole area of treatment for GH deficiency is now being explored in clinical trials—growth hormone releasing hormone (GHRH). This releasing hormone normally produced by the hypothalamus is, after all, the one that gets the pituitary to release GH. Maybe an extra dose would get the pituitary going. If this worked and the pituitary responded, then the natural GH might be released on the normal pituitary schedule which is so hard to mimic by injection.

In 1985 Michael Thorner and other researchers at the University of Virginia reported the treatment of GH-deficient children with biosynthetic GHRH, infusing them one minute every three hours by means of an infusion pump through a catheter. A change in body composition consistent with a rise in GH was noticed in the first week of treatment. In the six months study one child went from a growth rate of 4.6 cm (1.81 inches) per year to a rate of 7.1 cm (2.8 inches) per year, and the other went from 2.1 cm. (.83 inch) to 13.7 cm (5.39 inches) per year. Other studies of treatment lasting six to 18 months have reported growth rates of 7 cm. (2.76 inches) to 10 cm. (3.9 inches) per year.

GHRH treatment in this particular case seems as effective as GH treatment. But it opens up a big question. If GH-deficiency is caused by pituitary damage, as the hypopituitary diagnosis suggests, how could an extra dose of GHRH help any more than more gas can make a broken engine run? The fact that GHRH treatment did stimulate GH production suggested that the origin of GH-deficiency may often be GHRH-deficiency, a dysfunction of the hypothalamus instead of the pituitary.

A research team at the University of California, San Francisco, used GHRH on five boys whose GH production had become deficient following radiation for leukemia. Their subsequent growth demonstrated that cranial radiation can lead to hypothalamic dysfunction, treatable with GHRH. Response to GHRH treatment has become a means to distinguishing between hypothalamic GH-deficiency and pituitary GH-deficiency.

"It now appears that the majority of children with GH deficiency have hypothalamic dysfunction rather than pituitary somatotroph dysfunction," said Thorner. Other researchers agree the level of hypothalamic involvement is about 95%.

Besides whatever advantages there may be in stimulating GH production at the hypothalamic level, there is one other possibility that may someday make GHRH therapy preferable to conventional GH therapy. Researchers are experimenting with a nasal delivery system for GHRH. Using normal adults, French researchers M. Colle et al. demonstrated that results of a puff of GHRH dissolved in water in each nostril were comparable with results of GH injection. GH itself is a very large molecule, much larger than GHRH, and therefore has a harder time getting into the blood stream. The chances of GHRH being nasally delivered for now are better than the chances that GH can be administered without injection.

In spite of these hopeful possibilities, studies on GHRH treatment since Thorner's have had mixed results. In general, recent studies show GHRH treatment to be inferior to those of GH treatment, though it is not understood why. There is hope that GHRH agonists, that is, effective substitutes, with even smaller molecules may be developed to permit intranasal treatment. More readily absorbed and longer acting, these agonists might well be cheaper, too.

Another avenue of treatment being explored is growth hormone releasing peptide (GHRP). Tulane scientist C. Bowers and associates synthesized a set of six- and seven-amino acid peptides that activate GH release by a mechanism different from that of GHRH. These compounds work through injection or oral administration. They may represent the future therapy of choice.

In the meantime, about 12,000 children in this country alone, who have been diagnosed as GH-deficient through tests or by growth response to GH, bravely take their GH injections daily, measure themselves, and hope.

One such child, Brent Carney, has a story of growth hormone treatment to tell that will stick in your mind long after you have forgotten the details of our grown-up description. Brent's story is our next chapter.

CHAPTER EIGHT

Brent's Story

Brent Carney is growth hormone-deficient. But he is lucky. Not only was he born at a time when GH replacement therapy was available, but he had alert and supportive parents, knowledgeable and experienced physicians, and a good medical plan. Brent's small size was first recognized as abnormal when he was two, and then... But the best way to learn Brent's story is to let him tell you. When he was nine, he wrote and illustrated (in color) his own story, which we are privileged to include (in black and white, alas) on the following pages.

SHORT STUFF!

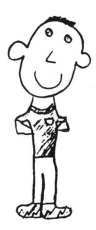

By: Brent Carney

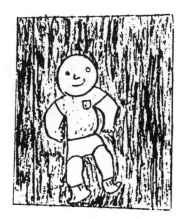

When I was born, I weighed 9 pounds and was 21 inches long. Until I was 3, I was big for my age. Then something happened. I started not to grow as much.

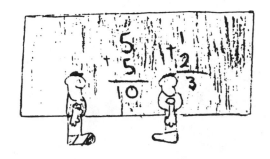

By the time I started
kindergarten I was shorter
than everybody. When I
went to the doctor she
said I would have a
growing spurt. Then, when
I was 6 years old I
went to a new doctor
and he said I would
grow when I was 8.

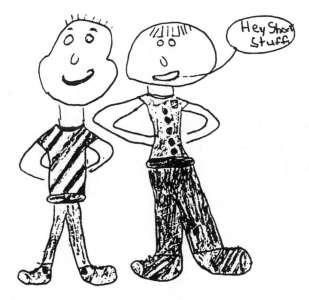

When I was 7 years old,
people were asking if I was
in kindergarten. One of my
friends used me for an arm
rest I was so short. Kids
culled me stuff like Short
Stuff, Shrimp and Chicken
Little. That really made
me sad. It hurt my
feelings.

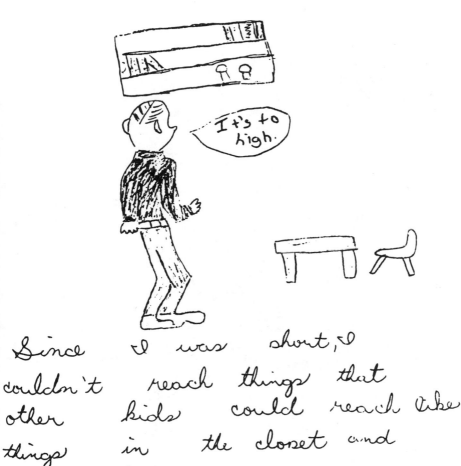

Since I was short, I couldn't reach things that other kids could reach like things in the closet and refrigerator.

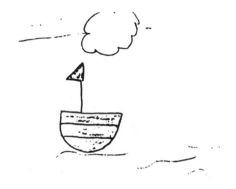

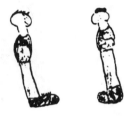

Sometimes I couldn't go on alot of rides at White Water. When I went to Pearl Harbor I was an inch short but they let me go on the boat anyway. My 4 year old brother was almost taller than me when I was 8.

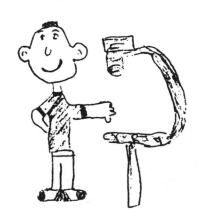
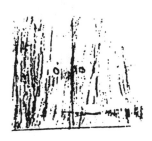

When I was eight, I went to
see a new doctor and she
said that I would have
to go see a special doctor
named Dr. Shultz, an endocrinologist. Dr. Shultz said I
would need to have an
Xray of my hand to see
what my bone age was.
My bone age was four and
remember I was eight at
the time.

151

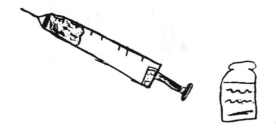

Dr. Shultz said that I will probably have to take shots to grow up but would have to wait until I am ten.

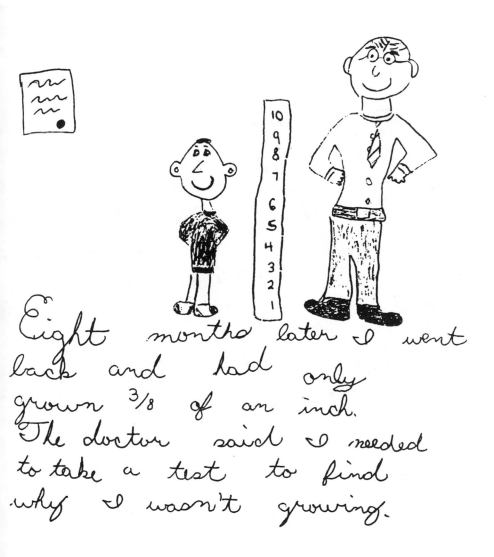

Eight months later I went back and had only grown 3/8 of an inch. The doctor said I needed to take a test to find why I wasn't growing.

When I took the test it took forever to find a vein. They stuck me three times and finally found a vein. The doctors had to put in a special needle because they thought it would fall out. I couldn't move my arm at all. The first thing they did was put L-Dopa through the needle. Every 30 minutes they took blood from my arm. They did this for 2 hours. Then they put Insulin through the needle. They drew blood every 30 minutes.

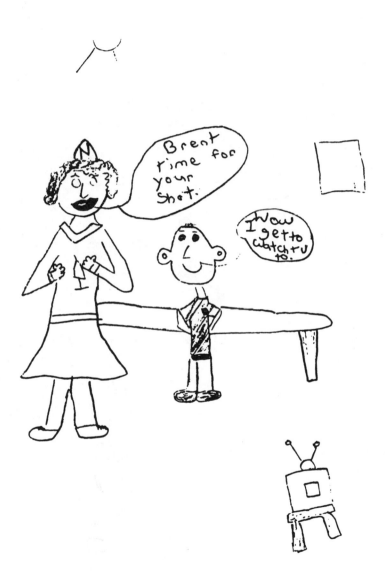

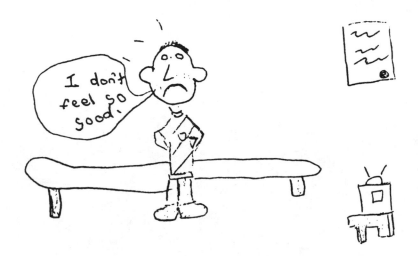

I got really hot and then went to sleep. When I woke up I was still sweaty and I got really sick. We had to stay there an hour longer because of me getting sick.

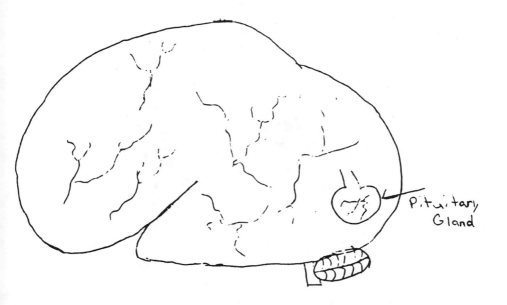

Pituitary
Gland

The test showed my
Pituitary Gland was
not working at all.
That is why I was
not growing. Now the
doctor said even though
I was not ten years
old yet, I could take
the shots.

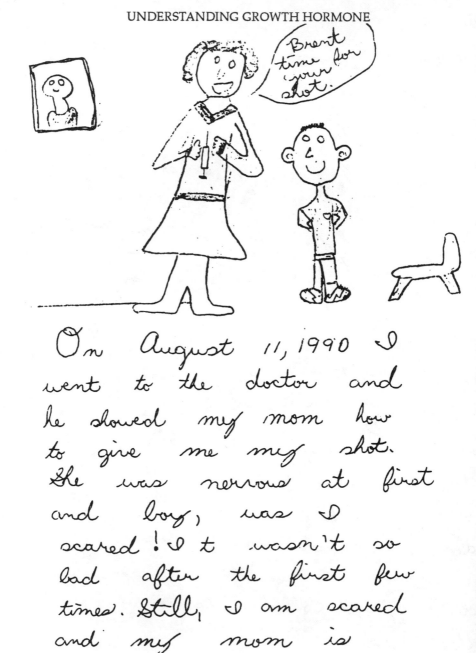

On August 11, 1990 I went to the doctor and he showed my mom how to give me my shot. She was nervous at first and boy, was I scared! It wasn't so bad after the first few times. Still, I am scared and my mom is nervous.

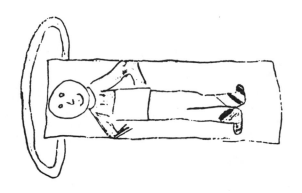

Right after we started the shots I had a CAT Scan to make sure I did not have a brain tumor blocking my Pituitary Gland. The CAT Scan was alright.

I got dizzy and they gave me a shot in in the foot and it hurt alot. Then they gave it to me in the other foot because they lost my vein. Then I was done.

The kind of shot I take is a synthetic growth hormone called Protropin I take shots every night before I go to bed. I will have to do this until I'm 17 years old.

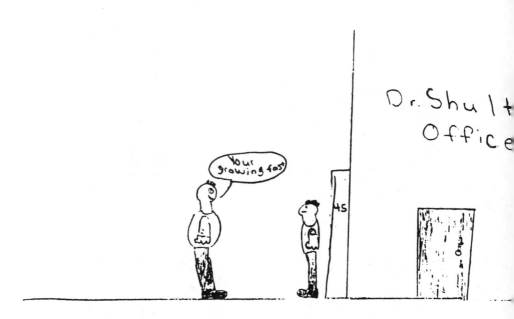

The first three months I grew 1⅝ inches. Dr. Shultz thought this was great. I also was getting skinnier.

I went back three months later, on February 14, 1941, and had grown 2 more inches. Dr. Shultz couldn't believe it. He told me that the first year expected growth was four to six inches. I had already grown 3 5/8 inches in six months. On February 18, 1941, I went for another bone age x-ray. My bone age now is six to seven years. ~~Soon~~ I will catch up with the other boys my age. I'll be glad of that.

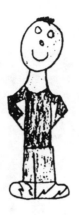

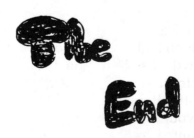

CHAPTER NINE

GH for More Short Kids?

In 1970 the Baxters had a baby boy seven weeks prematurely. Little Scott weighed just under five pounds at birth and measured 17 inches long. The pediatrician predicted, "In time he will catch up."

But in what time? Scott grew steadily but slowly and by school age was the size of a two-year-old. The Baxters held him back a year in school, but he was still smaller than his classmates. He began to ask, "When am I going to grow?" His parents wondered about the same question.

When Scott was ten, they heard about a doctor in another city who had treated a lot of children successfully for growth disorders and they went to consult him. This doctor told them that growth hormone might not make Scott taller as an adult than he would have been but it would make him grow right now. That's what they wanted to hear because they were tired of waiting.

When they told their pediatrician they were going to have Scott treated with GH, the pediatrician said, "I'm not going to speak to you again," and marched out of the room. The Baxters began to take Scott for treatment to an out-of-town endocrinologist—and found another pediatrician.

Scott began to grow faster. The Baxters feel the growth at that time was important in relieving anxiety—Scott's and theirs—and developing self-esteem. Scott is now twenty-one years old and a comfortable 5 feet 8. His parents will never know how tall he would have been without GH—maybe the same, maybe shorter, maybe taller.

The Baxters consider Scott's treatment a success story; critics consider the treatment unnecessary, possibly harmful, also expensive, painful, and probably unethical. It must be noted that in a time when GH was limited in supply and reserved for GH-deficient children, Scott Baxter, to his parents' knowledge, was never diagnosed as GH-deficient.

Scott's condition passed more than one expert's definition of GH-deficiency, however. David B. Allen and Norman C. Fost of the University of Wisconsin School of Medicine have said in a 1990 article, "First, there is no clear boundary between GH deficiency and sufficiency. Responses to stimulation tests do not mirror endogenous GH secretion. A continuum of 'inadequate' GH secretion spans classically and partially GH-deficient children, children with constitutional growth and pubertal delay, and other poorly growing short children who pass provocative tests but nevertheless secrete less GH than their peers. Thus a poorly growing child who achieves a normal growth rate with GH therapy would meet a functional definition of GH 'insufficiency' regardless of diagnostic test results."

But this definition—that GH works—called "an extreme view" by Emory's Parks, may also be applied to forms of short stature clearly or, at least, traditionally not related to GH-deficiency. This is where the battle lines are drawn.

Two Sides to the Issue

If GH makes kids grow, why don't we give all short children GH? There are two answers given by conservative researchers, physicians, and the FDA. One involves efficacy (Does the drug work?), and the other pertains to safety (Does the drug do any harm?).

First, conservative physicians say GH treatment might work temporarily but it has not been proven to make non-GH-deficient kids grow taller than they would otherwise grow. Short kids of many different kinds may have growth spurts when GH treatment begins, but they may slow down and finally stop growing at the height they would have grown untreated. Treatment with synthetic GH at optimum dosage and frequency is so new that too few children treated have reached the end of their growing years to judge efficacy. There is also evidence of "catch-down" growth, when kids who have taken GH grow more slowly after treatment stops than they did before treatment as if seeking an inevitable height.

But, more liberal doctors argue that even if the end gain is negligible, growth *now* will bring the kids closer to their age mates during the critical time when they are most vulnerable to being different, when their self-esteem is in the formative stages. Conservatives argue that measures of achievement and adjustment have never shown that short children suffer from their short stature. It is largely parents who project their own view that shortness is a problem on their kids—"Doctors and lawyers, mostly...," says one pediatric endocrinologist.

As for efficacy, say the liberals, GH is bound to work. "HGH given in sufficient dosages for long enough must increase final height," says researcher F. Darende-liler of Middlesex Hospital in London. "If it did not do so, tall adults in general and pituitary giants in particular would not exist."

Aye, there's the rub. Pituitary giants certainly prove the efficacy of GH, but pituitary giants generally die an early death, having suffered consequences of their excess from diabetes to arterial and cardiac degeneration. Emory endocrinologist Christy says, "In GH deficiency it's natural to replace the GH just as you replace thyroid or estrogen, but to do so in the absence of deficiency is very dangerous. Think what it can do to their arterial system and to their heart tissue." Endocrinologists like Christy see the ravages of acromegaly often. Pediatric endocrinologists do not. The closer the doctor is to acromegaly, the more likely he is to hold the conservative view that GH must never be given to a patient who does not demonstrate GH-deficiency on a standard test.

The Controversy

The controversy over whether to give GH to children who do not test GH-deficient began before synthesis of GH when some doctors put short patients on GH regardless of their GH-status. The scarcity of the natural hormone spawned ethical dilemmas over who should get the substance and who would be denied.

Surfeit, however, spawned its own set of ethical dilemmas as was evident from about 1986 when drug manufacturer Genentech first caught up with the demand for Protropin, the first synthetic GH approved by the FDA the year before. In an oft cited article by Gina Kolata in the October 1986 issue of *Science*, Tanner was quoted as saying, " We are now moving from an era in which there were too many patients chasing too little growth hormone to an era in which there will be too much growth hormone chasing too few patients."

While the article mentioned the elderly and the obese as possible quarry in the chase, the first widespread cross-over or "off-label" use (that is, a use not printed on the label of the drug) would be for short children not GH-deficient. "Growth hormone treatment," Tanner told *Science*'s Kolata, "may well become as accepted as orthodontia." Predicting what groups of people might one day be taking GH as a matter of course, he added, "It is really Brave New World." Emory's John Parks derisively dubbed the anticipated casual use of GH "cosmetic endocrinology."

The *Science* article also expressed researchers' fears that "the hormone will never be properly tested in clinical trials." A few paragraphs were devoted to the likelihood that a flood of research would probably bypass proper placebo-controlled clinical treatment to test efficacy. In historical studies comparing the growth of currently treated subjects with the growth of similar subjects in a time before the treatment in question was available, the possibility exists that the attention kids get or optimism or some other unrecognized factor to which experimental subjects are exposed is the real growth-promoting element. After all, if emotional neglect can cause kids to stop growing, an intense interest by a kindly research team might promote growth. The reluctance to use a double blind experiment for long term GH treatment is, of course, that if GH treatment does prove effective long term, those short children on the placebo will have missed the chance for treatment during their critical years. How many parents would want their kids to take years of shots for a 50% chance of getting nothing?

The *Science* article ends with Tanner's wistful remark

about GH therapy, "...all of us, in our hearts, believe it will work. But, in many ways, I rather think it would be better if it did not."

Five years and much research later (some of it not placebo controlled), on non-GH-deficient children, the controversy still rages. In June 1991, the *New York Times Magazine* ran a feature about the use of GH with short children that seemed to say the earlier fears had come true. Author Barry Werth focused on eleven-year-old Marco Oriti, who for his whole life has been several inches shorter than average and had a predicted adult height of 5 feet 4 inches—an often normal height shared by many famous people—but not what the typical all-American boy wants to achieve. This article repeated the Brave New World quote from Tanner, noted the pressure on researchers and academics to be on the cutting edge of research in new areas, and cited the profit-motive of drug companies to expand the use of the drug. The article also explained that most kids in the shortest three percentiles of height are normal—normally short. If these kids were treated so that none of them has to endure being that short, then the next three percentiles would become the unacceptably short, and so on.

This kind of article angers parents of children with verified GH-deficiency. The Horners' son has taken GH since the age of two. The Horner family is not dealing with the bottom three percentiles; they are talking about an off-the-chart growth deficit and severe illness as a result of multi-hypopituitarism. Without GH their son would probably reach an adult height of not much more than 4 feet. Hormone replacement is controlling most of the child's problems and the Horners expect their child, with the help of GH therapy, to reach his genetic limit as an adult. "Why don't they write about that?" asks Nadine Horner.

"Why don't they write about the good growth hormone does for children like ours? Why do they have to look for the negative?" The Horners are angry because the focus of the press is on the normal children and parents who are driven to GH by vanity and the desire for a competitive edge rather than relief from a disease. From such articles the public gets a generally negative view of GH, of the doctors who prescribe it, and of its uses. Negative publicity fuels insurance companies' reluctance to pay for GH treatment. It does a disservice to those children who really need it, say the Horners.

In 1990 several parents of GH-deficient children were interviewed at length by CNN about their experience with GH therapy and their participation in a screening for growth problems at a local health center. The parents told their story, emphasizing the need for public awareness. "Pediatricians are slow to acknowledge failure to grow and some children do not get much needed treatment for serious disorders as soon as they should," said one parent. Subsequently, CNN aired a documentary segment that the parents say focused primarily on misuse of GH. None of the remarks of the parents of GH-deficient children were included. "There will always be some instances of abuse of any substance but why focus on that and omit the good?" one frustrated parent asks.

"The press," agrees Kim Frye, director of chapter development for the Human Growth Foundation, "makes it look like GH is something parents want to give their kids for cosmetic reasons or to make their child into a basketball player. I resent that. GH is very expensive, we have to worry about keeping it cold everywhere we go, injections hurt, it's not fun. Very,

very few parents would do all that if they didn't have to. If they are going to show the side of misuse, why don't they also show the children who are receiving GH because of medical necessity?"

The distance between parents of hormone-deficient children and parents of children like Marco Oriti, who just wants to be taller, may seem simple. On the one hand we have children with a disease, on the other hand children who are well. What is not so simple is that there is a whole spectrum of children who are abnormally short and do suffer from a disease but, not testing as GH-deficient, are not classic candidates for GH. Physicians are nevertheless trying GH therapy on many categories of growth-retarding diseases in research protocols, that is, experimental studies approved by the FDA. Truly abnormal and absolved from the sin of vanity, these groups of short children still face the questions of efficacy and safety of GH *for them.*

Turner Syndrome: A Case in Point

A disorder that is challenging our understanding of GH and how it works is Turner Syndrome. Its successful treatment with GH is breaking medical barriers for non-GH deficient, abnormally short children.

Turner Syndrome is a relatively common cause of growth failure afflicting about 50,000 girls in the United States or one in about 2,000 female births. In Turner Syndrome, an abnormality of the X (female) chromosome is associated with short stature, non-functional ovaries, and a variety of disturbances of the skeleton and other organs. While possible symptoms of Turner Syndrome fill a whole page of a medical book, a particular Turner patient may have only one or two of the signs. Growth disruption, present in 95% of those afflicted, is often the first visible sign of the disease. A karyotype, as a chromosome test which can identify Turner Syndrome is called, should be done for any girl with unexplained short stature. GH therapy today is considered to be appropriate treatment for girls with Turner, although this use of the hormone had not yet been approved by the FDA as of July 1992.

In Coral Springs, Florida, Danielle, a young girl diagnosed with Turner Syndrome, is being treated with GH. As a toddler Danielle was tiny but growing at a steady rate. Her mother, Jeannie, is only 4 feet 11, her father, Frank, only 5 feet 7. Because her parents were small, no one thought to evaluate Danielle for a growth disorder. At age four, Danielle was taken to a new pediatrician for bronchitis. The doctor on call, not her regular pediatrician, noticed a telltale extra fold of skin on the back of Danielle's neck which is a sign of Turner Syndrome. When tests verified the diagnosis, Danielle's parents were offered GH treatment for her. At that time, synthetic GH was relatively new, and, since Danielle was still growing at a normal rate, they decided to wait and watch. Three years later Danielle's growth had dropped below a normal rate. She was, as so many short kids' parents say, "off the chart," and Danielle's parents knew the time for treatment had come.

Danielle was delighted to be on GH at first, "a real trooper," her mom says, at taking the injections. After a month, however, the novelty had worn off and Danielle rebelled. Her parents put stickers on her special calendar and gave her treats for good behavior, but nothing worked. An injection that should have taken ten seconds was taking an hour.

"We had to take the tension out of the house," says Jeannie. They decided to take Danielle to the pediatrician's office every day for her shots. "The first day there was an argument," Jeannie recalls. "The second day there was a fight, the third day there was a temper tantrum. On the fourth day, Danielle said, 'I don't want to go to the doctors office anymore. I want you to give me my medicine at home.'" She had accepted the necessity, as most patients do. Three years later Danielle goes to the homes of other growth deficient children beginning GH treatment and teaches families how to give and take injections.

At eleven years, ten months, Danielle is now 4 feet 3 inches, near the fifth percentile. "It was so great at Christmas to see Danielle singing in a chorus on the front row and there were three other children the same size as she is. She's done great," says Jeannie.

Danielle will stay on GH until she reaches "a normal height," say her parents. "We're not looking for the jolly green giant. We just want her to be able to drive a car, function normally, and feel good about herself."

Turner Syndrome success stories sound a lot like GH-deficiency success stories but there are differences. In the first studies, when Turner girls were given GH three times a week, their growth rate did not increase as much as the growth of GH-deficient children had. Even today gains are modest compared to GH-deficiency cases, which represent a greater degree of growth failure. From historical data, the projected mean height for a Turner girl was about 142 centimeters or 4 feet 8. The majority of Turner patients started on GH treatment in 1983, according to R.G. Rosenfeld of the Stanford University Department of Pediatrics, have passed this mark and are still growing. A final mean height of 150 cm. or 4 feet 11 inches is anticipated. Those extra few inches make the difference between perceived dwarfism and normal height. The early gain in height with GH treatment also allows doctors to induce puberty (and, consequently, growth plate closure) with estrogen at a more appropriate age.

Turner Syndrome is interesting because it represents a growth disorder successfully treated by GH but not generally considered to be based on GH-deficiency. Since GH production is known to be higher in the presence of estrogen and since one aspect of Turner Syndrome is lack of estrogen production, it seems logical that Turner Syndrome girls might lack GH. In fact, some Turner girls (including Danielle) test on the low end of the normal scale, and some are clearly deficient. Most Turner girls, however, do not test positive for GH-deficiency. There is still debate about whether the GH secretory status of Turner Syndrome patients contributes to their growth failure.

Toshiaki Tanaka of the National Children's Hospital in Japan and his colleagues shed light on the question in a 1991 report of a study of 151 young patients with Turner Syndrome. The Japanese researchers tested the GH secretion of all the patients by more than two different stimulation tests, dividing them into categories: Complete GH-deficiency was defined as the status of patients with less than 7 ng/ml of peak GH; partial GH-deficiency was defined as the status of patients who had between 7 and 10 ng/ml of peak GH; those with 10 or more ng/ml were considered normal. In fact, 10% of the patients were completely GH-deficient; another 10% were partially deficient; and 80% had normal GH secretion. The 20% with some degree of GH-deficiency is too low to say GH-deficiency causes the growth failure in Turner Syndrome, but too high to ignore. However, mean peak GH secretion in this study did not correlate significantly with growth velocity or how the subjects compared in height to others of their age. Tanaka concluded that GH secretion capacity in

Turner Syndrome does not affect growth. These researchers subsequently treated the girls with GH and the growth of all three groups accelerated. GH treatment, says Tanaka, did not provide replacement GH but had another pharmacological effect.

In the United States, when GH provocation tests have yielded normal, even low normal results, Turner patients have not officially been considered GH-deficient. GH treatment for Turner Syndrome has not been FDA approved, and the treatment has been considered investigational. Since physicians are allowed, using their own judgment, to prescribe GH anyway—it is, after all, a legal drug—the main problem may lie with insurance coverage.

The company that insured Danielle's family through a group plan at Frank's work paid for her initial GH when her endocrinologist prescribed treatment. But, because of skyrocketing insurance premiums, Frank's employer sought alternative insurance. After being assured the new policy would guarantee coverage for Danielle and her GH treatment, the employer changed companies. A few months later, when a claim was filed, Danielle was denied. Since then the group was dissolved and Danielle's parents were told to seek individual coverage. It was then learned Danielle was uninsurable and had no alternative but to be placed on a state comprehensive plan. GH, approved for GH inadequacy, is considered by some to be experimental for girls with Turner Syndrome. Danielle is doing very well on GH therapy and her family is waiting for the expected FDA approval they feel will help many girls with Turner Syndrome.

Danielle's story is not unusual, but certainly many insurance companies look at more than just the numbers on the GH tests. They look at the growth charts, too. If a child is growing suboptimally, some companies will approve payment for GH treatment. They will then track growth and approve treatment as long as it is getting good results.

The slowness of the FDA to approve an accepted treatment is one factor that can hinder treatment. Another factor can be public opinion, as was demonstrated by another setback for Turner Syndrome therapy. Some investigators had reported that treatment with GH and the anabolic steroid oxandrolone was even better than with either treatment alone. In particular, Rosenfeld studied 65 patients with Turner Syndrome treating them with GH alone, oxandrolone alone, and a combination of GH and oxandrolone together. The GH treatment was effective, doubling the rate of growth over the control group and increasing the projected adult height by 4.5 cm. The oxandrolone treatment alone gave similar or better results than the GH treatment. The combined GH/oxandrolone treatment was the best, tripling the untreated growth rate and increasing the projected height by 8.2 cm. No undesirable side effects were reported.

Unfortunately, there was so much adverse publicity associated with anabolic steroids during the 1988 Olympics that the American manufacturer of oxandrolone at that time, G.D. Searle Co., withdrew its product, Anavar (R), from the market. This is an example of misuse of a drug making the drug suspect for all—even legitimate—purposes. This is the pattern that parents of abnormally short children fear for GH. For several years GH alone remained the best treatment for growth retardation in Turner Syndrome. Then, in the last months of 1991, another pharmaceutical company, Gynex, under an arrangement with Searle, began offering an oxandrolone product called Oxandrin (R), re-opening the possibility of combined treatment.

GH therapy for Turner Syndrome in spite of these difficulties has progressed from a faint possibility to the never-never land of wide use without FDA approval and will probably soon win FDA approval and a more favorable treatment by insurance companies. This long journey may be a preview of what is to come in the field of GH therapy for other non-GH-deficient disorders.

One might ask if the successful treatment of Turner Syndrome with GH is a way of saying that GH status does not matter. Or that values for low GH are set too low. Or that the body can tolerate some degree of GH that is supraphysiological, that is, more than natural. The answers to these questions must be determined for each disorder, one by one.

Other Kinds of Short Stature: Is GH Treatment a Possibility?

Whatever the GH status, ever since the availability of GH, some consideration has been given by some investigators to treat each of the other growth disorders with GH. Experimental treatment has been conducted for many disorders as well as for normal subjects. Experimental and anecdotal results have varied over the years.

In 1989 Darendeliler summarized the state of the art using published and unpublished data from colleagues in research on non-conventional uses of GH in Europe. Darendeliler concluded, "It is evident from these studies that hGH is far more successful in promoting growth in a variety of conditions than earlier reports suggested. The better response is probably due to more frequent administration of GH in doses appropriate for body size." Although the question of ultimate height of these patients still remains, he notes that all children respond to GH with an increased growth rate.

German researcher J.R.Bierich, of the University of Tubingen Department of Pediatrics, points out not only that GH is effective in a number of non-GH deficient kinds of short stature but that more of these disorders than previously thought do have a GH connection.

Here is a run-down of short stature categories by cause from the normal to the abnormal with a summary of findings about treatment and GH status.

Chip Off the Old Block: Familial Short Stature

Arturo at age sixteen is 5 feet 3. He is waiting to grow taller. He will wait in vain because his mother is barely 5 feet tall and his father is 5 feet 2 1/2. Few of his aunts and uncles are much taller. Arturo has been growing steadily and, like most kids of his generation, is already taller than his same-sex parent. Though he is shorter than most of the guys at school, he's as tall as the genes he got from his parents will allow. Arturo's small size is called *familial short stature*. That is the term used when a healthy child from a short family is at or below the fifth percentile on the growth chart. Somebody has to be smallest, right? The condition is perfectly normal, and one would wish, completely acceptable. Arturo, however, is still unhappy with his lot.

Do Arturo and other normal short children have less GH than their taller peers? Is GH production the key to stature even for normal people? The relationship between normal growth and GH production has not been conclusively studied. Statements from some experts reflect their belief that there is a relationship, but some studies have found no relationship between GH production and height or bone age among children of normal height. An alternative theory is that the critical hereditary component is the degree of sensitivity of the target organs to stimulation by GH or to the growth factor next in line on the chain of endocrine command, Sm-C/IGF-I.

Whether short children from short families could be treated with GH and grow taller is still the $64,000 question. (Or $164,000 question because that's how much ten years of GH could cost.)Darendeliler says, "Trials of therapy in children growing slowly, whatever their GH response to provocative stimuli, do not address the crucial issue for which an answer is demanded by society which is whether adult stature of normal individuals can be increased by hGH and what are the implications of the treatment."

In a 1984 study of short normal children conducted by J.M. Gertner and others from Yale and Stanford, all ten subjects given GH three times a week for six months showed an increase in growth velocity; even the smallest absolute increment of 1.2 cm/yr represented a growth velocity 33% higher than that observed before treatment. No adverse results were detected. Other investigators have found little or no growth increase. Daniel Rudman had earlier found a subset of normal children with short stature who did respond to GH, suggesting that there may be different bases for short stature among so-called normal children. There have actually been relatively few trials on short normals, and those few have not been conducted long enough to be conclusive. Trials conducted before 1985, moreover, did not have the benefit of unlimited supplies of biosynthetic GH and the new dosage/frequency schedules now used. Barbara Linder and Fernando Cassoria, speaking of studies reported in 1981-1983, said, "Initial studies have been encouraging in that many of these children will grow faster with short-term growth hormone use. Whether this increased height velocity can be sustained without deleterious advancement in bone age or other potential side effects remains to be determined by long-term, controlled studies."

Research may go on, but familial short stature is probably the one area where the most experts will object to the use of GH as not medically indicated and therefore unethical, truly "cosmetic endocrinology." The majority view is expressed by John Lantos and Mark Siegler of the Center for Clinical Medical Ethics, and Leona Cuttler of the Pediatric Endocrinology section at the University of Chicago Pritzker School of Medicine: "For children who are relatively short but have no documented GH abnormality, normal growth velocity, and predicted adult height above the fifth percentile, we suggest that GH therapy is not routinely indicated. This condition does not fit any current concept of a disease state, there is no evidence that such children are at risk for psychosocial morbidity, and their appearance would not be so abnormal that burdensome and potentially risky cosmetic therapy would be justified." Psychological counseling has been suggested as a far better approach to easing the discomfort of short normal children than any kind of growth therapy.

Speaking to pediatricians about the use of GH for relief from the pressures of cultural prejudice, Lantos et al. said, "If pediatricians do not respond to these dilemmas thoughtfully, carefully, and forcefully, other decision makers, whose decisions may reflect political, social, or market forces, may then respond in ways that do not reflect the best interests of children."

Too Little Too Late: Growth Delay

Shawn was almost fourteen and 4 feet 7 inches. Most of the boys in his class at school were well over 5 feet and many were quite developed. Shawn looked like a little boy beside his friends, some of whom were already shaving occasionally. The girls towered over Shawn and he wouldn't think of asking one of them to dance. Shawn's parents were average height, and they were also worried. Shawn seemed perfectly healthy, but why was he so short?

Actually, Shawn is expected to reach a normal height of 5 feet 9 inches; it's just going to take a while to get there. He is growing steadily but a little less every year than his friends and he is a couple years later than average reaching puberty. A pediatric endocrinologist, who evaluated Shawn's case, has said Shawn has *constitutional delay of growth and adolescence*. The physician does not worry that Shawn will end up abnormally short because he has X-rayed Shawn's bones and determined that his bone age is also equally delayed. His growth plates are as open as an eleven-year-old's and he has several more years of growing to do, more years than his friends who have already entered puberty. Shawn is what is known as a late-bloomer. How did the doctor know? While giving the doctor his family history, Shawn's father recalled that he himself had been the smallest boy in the class for most of his school years; then as a late teenager had shot up to a height of 5 feet 11 inches. A family history of late-blooming can help the doctor diagnose the situation correctly.

Constitutional delay of growth and adolescence is seen far more often in boys than in girls. Treatment is not often recommended, especially for girls. Delayed maturity and short stature negatively affect the self-esteem of adolescent boys far more than girls. In a 1979 study by F. Douglas Frasier, 90 to 95% of the children whose parents expressed concern about their growth were boys with constitutional growth delay.

Constitutional delay of growth and adolescence is often listed as a normal variation in growth because children with this delay seem healthy and they often reach the mid-parental height.

Not all investigators agree, however, that constitutional delay of growth and adolescence is a normal delay, especially as some children with delayed growth and adolescence do end up shorter than predicted by their parents' height. Such children when measured by provocative GH tests have typically shown normal results, are not considered GH-deficient, and therefore have not been treated with GH. However, says German investigator Bierich, citing studies from 1983 to 1987, measurement of spontaneous GH secretion shows that relatively low GH production, about 50% of the mean, is indeed the cause of the delay. Bierich concludes that, "If the slow growth of the patients is due to diminished GH secretion, then treatment by GH is replacement therapy."

Emory University's John Parks does not buy Bierich's reasoning. GH secretion increases with puberty, Parks reiterates. Most short boys with delayed adolescence are therefore going to be low in GH compared to other fourteen-year-old boys by reason of their delayed puberty, but their time will come. GH will rise and a growth spurt will happen for these late bloomers.

Bierich has tried GH therapy, nonetheless, with subjects with delayed growth and adolescence. In Bierich's first such study in 1983, he achieved an average growth velocity increase of 100%. Similar trials by different investigators using one year of treatment corroborated Bierich's conclusion. A four-year study by Bierich, published in 1986, shows "classic catch-up growth." It is still uncertain whether the adult height was taller than it would have been in time without treatment.

The question remains concerning the importance of growth now when weighed against the uncertainty of GH treatment. We have heard from parents and patients who think growth now is enormously important. If it seems so critical, Parks conservatively recommends, "Give delayed puberty boys testosterone and girls estrogen to bring on puberty and the growth spurt. Treatment with sex hormones costs only a fraction of what GH costs and it is known to be safe."

In fact, that is what Shawn's pediatric endocrinologist recommended. He has had four injections of testosterone and already he is growing faster, his body is changing, and he looks a little less like a little kid.

Little Acorns: Intrauterine Growth Retardation

David Sanders was born full term weighing five pounds two ounces and measuring 17 inches long. He was cute, perfectly formed, small-boned, and plump. In the first weeks after birth, he neither lost weight nor gained weight, then he started steady but slow growth. The pediatrician tried changing formulas and pushing solid food to no avail. The baby smiled his way to toddlerhood, however, and his small size, at the fifth percentile, was not considered a problem at that time. At the age of one, his parents discovered David was deaf. His mother had been exposed to rubella or German measles, during pregnancy, although no rash was observed, and a test of David's blood showed David also had been exposed to German measles. Apparently, rubella had damaged the baby's hearing before birth. After data from a rubella epidemic that year had been analyzed, it was noted that babies, particularly boy babies, with pre-natal rubella damage were on the average smaller in stature from birth to adulthood. David ultimately reached an adult height of 5 feet 5 inches, five inches shorter than his brothers' heights and he remains very small-boned.

A full-term baby like David, born small with a length significantly under the average of 20 inches who does not grow at a normal rate, is said to have *intrauterine growth retardation* (IUGR). The baby may have suffered some infection, trauma, or nutritional deficiency in the uterus. Often the cause is not known. About half of these short babies catch-up in length by age two or three.

Studies in the 1970s of GH treatment for these born-small kids were disappointing. Trials in 1974 and 1979, however, showed a doubling of growth rate for two-thirds of the patients with IUGR. Again, the more favorable results are attributed to the doses and frequencies of GH injection used in the more recent studies, totaling more GH per week than earlier studies. Again, ultimate height comparisons are not available.

In a recent experiment, R. Stanhope of the Institute of Child Health in London studied children with low birth weight. GH treatment in higher than standard doses increased their growth but bone age advancement was disproportionately greater than the added height. For example, a seven-year-old child, several inches shorter than normal since birth, had a growth rate and bone maturity appropriate for his age. All he needed to do was make up the deficit he had been born with. Given GH, his growth rate increased but his bones began to mature even more rapidly. At the end of the first year of treatment, he was 4.25 inches taller but his growth plates were 1.75 years closer to closing than before. Obviously, if GH treatment were continued, immediate growth might be increased but the time growth was possible would be shortened, for a probable net loss.

Systemic Disease

Systemic disease, an illness that affects the whole body, may cause growth arrest. *Gastro-intestinal disease*, for example, is a common problem: Wayne was a lively two-year-old until he got the "flu." After most of his symptoms were gone, he was still lethargic. Also, he stopped digesting his food: Apple sauce went in and came out looking like fresh apple sauce; spinach, carrots and meat passed through unchanged. This went on for months during which Wayne lost weight and did not grow taller. Wayne's digestive system for some reason could not absorb the food normally or could not keep the food long enough to absorb it. The results were the same as starving. After many changes of diet, he recovered and then experienced a spurt of catch-up growth. An Italian endocrinology clinic examined by biopsy the duodenal (from the small intestine) tissue of 60 children referred for short stature. Of these, 8.3% had signs of intestinal disease, passing food without digesting it, even though they had made no complaint about digestive problems. An English study found 25% of kids with short stature of unknown origin had digestive disorders. Growth for these children improved on a gluten-free diet.

Diseases like anemia, diabetes, lung disease, cystic fibrosis, heart disease may also be obstacles to normal growth. Kidney disease in particular has a negative effect on growth. Chronic renal (kidney) insufficiency retards skeletal growth, and, after successful treatment or transplant, catch-up growth rarely occurs. Are these kidney patients GH-deficient? Hardly. To the contrary, researchers uniformly report high levels of GH in patients with kidney disease. One explanation for resistance to the growth promoting effects of high GH is that abnormally high concentrations of a binding protein for Sm-C/IGF-I ties up the growth factor in the blood and keeps its growth-promoting activity away from cartilage cells. Researchers have been wary about giving exogenous GH to a patient whose GH is already high; nevertheless, experimental treatment with GH to increase SM-C/IGF-I to useful levels is in progress. Preliminary results in studies in the U.S. and in Europe show increased growth for those treated, justifying hopes that ultimately GH will improve the prospects of greater height in children with chronic kidney disease. Although increased GH may well overpower the binding problem, the direct action of the extra GH over a long period of time may prove to be excessive, to cause symptoms of acromegaly, or to worsen kidney function.

Hormone Disorders

GH-deficiency is just one endocrine disease that can disrupt growth. Another hormone insufficiency is hypothyroidism in which the thyroid gland does not produce enough hormone, especially thyroxine. Thyroid insufficiency before and shortly after birth causes cretinism, a condition in which short stature is often accompanied by mental retardation, deafness, and other abnormalities. Acquired hypothyroidism after age two or three is most often caused by an autoimmune disease of the thyroid called Hashimoto's Disease. Hypothyroidism at any stage of childhood will likely cause growth to slow or stop and bone age to slow. The deficiency may come on gradually and growth delay may be the first warning. Early detection is important because the degree of catch-up growth after treatment with thyroxin depends on how severe the hypothyroidism has been and how long the condition has existed.

Too much of a hormone can also cause a growth delay. For example, both Cushing's disease and an adrenal tumor can make the adrenal glands produce too much cortisol. The most common cause of excess cortisol in children, however, is a medicine containing cortisol prescribed for asthma or other disorder. Ryan, for example, had such bad asthma attacks that he was taken to the hospital emergency room 47 times the year he was eleven. His medication helped but the high doses of cortisol suppressed his GH production and impaired his growth. When this kind of medication is discontinued, catch-up growth depends on the degree and duration of the excess. Bierich has concluded in cases of long-term treatment by cortisol that GH treatment is justified. However, studies by Barbara Linder and associates from the National Institutes of Health in 1988 showed that treating with cortisol every other day is just as effective against asthma, etc., as daily doses but does not suppress GH. This remedy will probably prove more useful and simpler than GH therapy for growth. Also, another non-steroid medication, gamma globulin, is being tried experimentally with apparent success in reducing the dosage of steroids needed to control asthma.

Another endocrine disorder causes precocious puberty. Andrea, for example, at age 8, shot up taller than her friends and began to experience pubertal changes. Being unprepared, she was frightened and embarrassed. Not only did her early development distress her, but her ultimate height was foreshortened as growth plates closed far too early. On top of everything else, she went from being too big and mature to being too little as an adult.

Darendeliler reports that the precocious puberty of nine girls has been arrested by endocrinological intervention at Middlesex Hospital in London. This measure alone was not expected to increase the girls' adult height because with the slowing of pubertal development the girls' GH fell also. Treatment with GH during the extra pre-pubertal time showed encouraging preliminary results. However, in a study completed in 1988, Penelope Manasco, M.D., and others from the National Institutes of Health showed that increased growth was possible without GH therapy. Manasco reversed one type of precocious puberty of 20 girls and six boys and thereby significantly improved their predicted height well into the normal range because the puberty-slowing treatment also slowed the advancement of bone age to 2.6 years over five years of treatment. As long as the growth rate of these children exceeds bone age advancement, however that is achieved, GH treatment is not necessary.

Genetic Disorders

Genetic or inherited disorders account for some cases of failure to grow at a normal rate. Among these are chromosome disorders, errors and omissions in the chromosomes, the genetic building blocks. Some chromosomal disorders inhibit growth. One example is Turner Syndrome discussed earlier. Turner Syndrome is fairly common, occurring in one out of every 2,000 to 2,500 girls.

Another genetic growth disorder, named Laron-type dwarfism for researcher Zvi Laron at Tel Aviv University, is very rare but interesting because the Laron dwarf appears to be GH-deficient but actually has higher than normal GH levels. Laron-type dwarfism is a recessive disorder found among certain ethnic groups, especially among so-called oriental Jews, that is, Jews of middle Eastern origin who have heavily intermarried. A gene deletion on one chromosome eliminates the receptor that is needed to recognize growth hormone. Consequently the liver does not produce enough of the GH-dependent growth factor, Sm-C/IGF-I, and skeletal growth is severely reduced. The hypothalamus receives feedback that Sm-C/IGF-I is low and cracks the whip on the pituitary again. But no matter how much GH is produced, in the GH-resistant Laron dwarf, no Sm-C/IGF-I will be produced. Naturally, treatment with exogenous GH would only make matters worse. The best treatment, not yet proven, may be injections of Sm-C/IGF-I directly. Growth would probably occur and GH production would settle down.

Skeletal dysplasias are a group of genetic disorders that cause very short stature with abnormal body proportions. In this type of dwarfism, cartilage/bone cells in certain limbs seem unable to grow. In *achondroplasia*, one of the most common genetic bone disorders, the child's body grows normally in length but the arms and legs remain short. The head may be large. The hobby shopkeeper in Chapter Six was this kind of dwarf. His size did not keep him from enjoying several lively careers or from having attractive children who were dwarfs also. In other skeletal dysplasias the spine may be disproportionately short. There is no commonly used growth therapy for skeletal dysplasia, although research in GH therapy has been conducted. Twenty disproportionate dwarfs suffering from hypochondroplasia and achondroplasia were treated with GH by

Darendeliler and associates. Preliminary reports after one year were encouraging. Increased growth occurred with no unwanted advance in bone age and no increase in the degree of disproportion. Other researchers have found that one kind of dysplasia responded to GH while others did not. Another potential treatment explored by Linder and Cassoria is to use hormones to delay puberty in the hope that a longer period of growth will enhance final height. But delaying puberty may also reduce the pubertal growth spurt normally accompanied by a GH peak and end up yielding no ultimate increase. A combination of delaying puberty and adding GH is a promising route to be explored further.

You Are What You Eat—Or Don't Eat

Malnutrition is a sad and common reason for insufficient growth around the world. The cure is obvious but not often possible. Even in our relatively affluent society, there is malnutrition in pockets of poverty, not necessarily for lack of quantity but from lack of quality of diet.

Occasionally malnutrition appears in the most affluent circles. Parks recalls the fourteen-year-old son of a well-to-do family who was brought to him for evaluation for a growth disorder. He was then the height of the average eight year old. First Parks took a dietary history:

Parks: What does he eat?
Mother: Spaghetti.
Parks: What does he eat for breakfast?
Mother: Spaghetti.
Parks: What does he eat for lunch?
Mother: Spaghetti.

Parks: Does he eat snacks?
Mother: Yes. Spaghetti.
Parks: How much spaghetti does he eat in a day?

Eventually Parks determined that the boy had a snack-pack can of Chef Boyardee Spaghetti Os each day from which he ate a few bites every now and then during the day—inadequate total calories as well as insufficient variety! This was truly a case of growth deficiency due to malnutrition.

Why!? The boy had choked on a hot dog when he was younger, his mother explained, and ever after had been afraid to eat anything other than the safe, soft Spaghetti Os. As part of the solution to the boy's malnutrition, the boy had to have psychological counseling to overcome his fear. For that reason the boy's case overlaps with the next category.

Psychosocial Dwarfism

Psychosocial dwarfism is a failure to grow for psychological reasons. "The child who steals food from siblings' plates, eats from the dog's bowl, gorges and vomits is probably expressing the syndrome of psychosocial dwarfism," says Parks, adding that extreme cases are rare. The disorder includes a wide spectrum of unhealthy eating behavior and most often begins in the second or third year of life. "If children learn to eat in a stressed situation, they are at risk."

Besides children with eating disorders, children who live in abusive or negligent homes or who suffer emotional deprivation often fail to grow even if well fed. GH has been found depressed in such children, but if they are taken from the poor environment to a better one, GH production returns to normal and catch-up growth occurs. The process works in reverse as well; a return to the poor environment slows growth. Treatment with GH is not an acceptable solution to psychosocial dwarfism; physicians, counselors, and social workers must seek improvement of the underlying psychosocial factors.

Anorexia Athletica

Another kind of malnutrition is seen in young athletes. Fima Lifshitz at North Shore University Hospital on Long Island identified and named the disorder *anorexia athletica* after seeing a number of youngsters whose growth slowed down about the time of expected puberty. These athletes simply do not take in enough calories to maintain their high level of exercise and to grow at the same time. The disorder is particularly common among young performers who feel pressure to stay trim, such as gymnasts, divers, and ballet dancers.

Other Syndromes

In recent years, since Turner Syndrome has been successfully treated with GH, physicians are beginning to take a closer look at other syndromes involving short stature. Sometimes evaluation of the anomalies as a syndrome obscures the possibility that the growth disorder itself could be a GH-deficiency. "We're seeing genetic syndromes," says pediatric endocrinologist Stephen Anderson, "where the short stature has previously been written off. Doctors say, 'Well, you're short. But you have Prater-Willi or Russell-Silver or some other syndrome.' And that explanation ended the evaluation. But we are finding that, along with their other symptoms, a lot of these kids have GH-deficiency which can be treated with GH."

Idiopathic Short Stature

The word *idiopathic* comes from the Greek word *idio*, which, loosely translated, means "one of a kind," and the Greek word *path*, meaning "disorder." Idiopathic short stature does not fit any category. Lab tests on children with idiopathic short stature show all other measures are normal. No reason can be found for these children falling below normal in height. This does not mean there is no reason. Note that it was a group of subjects previously identified as examples of idiopathic short stature who exhibited a high rate of intestinal problems during a screening for digestive disease. In any case, *idio* is the prefix doctors use to mean "I dunno."

Between Caution and Risk

As more research is done on growth disorders, the question of treatment, including expanded use of GH becomes no less controversial. For every new answer there is a new question—and a new opinion:

Allen and Fost conclude, "In anticipation of more widespread use of GH, we argue that (1) GH responsiveness, not GH deficiency, should be a criterion for GH therapy; (2) the primary goal of GH therapy should be to alleviate the handicap of short stature rather than the treatment of GH deficiency; and (3) responsible distribution of and reimbursement for GH therapy should be guided by criteria of GH responsiveness and handicap, and not by a child's diagnosis." Allen and Fost have drawn a startling line in the sand based solely on how short the child is. The Wisconsin researchers say, "it is appropriate to restrict access, even within the group of GH-responsive children. As a starting point, we propose that treatment be limited to those for whom height is not merely a relative disadvantage but a serious handicap, arbitrarily defined as below the 1st percentile."

Allen and Fost add one cautionary—and more conventional—note to clinical physicians, "While costs are high, benefits unclear, and toxic effects uncertain, prescribing GH for non-GH deficient children outside of research protocols should be resisted."

We hope to have presented a balanced view of GH treatment by including what has been labeled the "extreme view" and the optimistic reviews of European researchers along with the conservative view of "no GH deficiency, no GH treatment" when GH deficiency means failing a stimulation test. With few exceptions, pediatric endocrinologists in clinical settings say they do not treat non-GH-deficient children with GH except for Turner cases; some, however, have been known to stretch the point.

As for a balanced summary of the field of GH treatment in short children, we cannot improve on that of UCLA's Barbara Lippe and S. Douglas Frasier in their 1989 overview in the *Journal of Pediatrics*, in which they reiterate that there are "no quick fixes in the realm of growth therapy."

The views of Lippe and Frasier should dampen the enthusiasm of short families for GH treatment for their short normal children. Their expert opinions should also allay the fears of alarmists who ask: If very short people can be made to grow, what about rather short people, or average people who want to be taller? Where would it all stop? Will it end with a society of two instantly recognizable socio-economic classes— the tall elite who can afford GH and the short underclass who can't get treatment? "Finally it should be pointed out," say Lippe and Frasier, as if in reply, "that even in the studies that do suggest a gain in final height, no improvement over calculated genetic height potential has been reported."

The UCLA researchers also emphasize that all children with abnormal shortness should be very thoroughly evaluated whether or not GH-deficiency is a factor. They acknowledge that GH treatment will sometimes be indicated in non-GH deficient cases and hopes that this will be done only for well-evaluated cases by qualified specialists only. Like Allen and Fost, Lippe and Frasier make the plea that the results of any non-traditional treatment not be lost to the larger research world. "If treatment of such children with GH is recommended, it should be administered either as a part of a prospective clinical trial or as an individual therapeutic trial designed to provide an on-going data base that can be used to direct subsequent therapeutic decisions."

A reasonable mix of caution and reasoned risk by those who have the most information and experience is what we should hope for. If everyone were cautious, and no one tried what was not yet proven, there would be no new treatment. Without someone willing to take the risks of the unknown, certainly, small stature as a part of Turner Syndrome would not now be treated. Who knows what disorder may be next?

Many have faulted drug companies for their efforts and support in broadening the use of GH as greedy, self-interested behavior. It must be said that corporate self-interest, that is to say, profit, has been the primary motive for producing some of the most magnificent boons to mankind—not a few of which have been drugs—as well as some unnecessary and even harmful products. We are left to trust in the integrity, education, and good judgment of the medical and research professions for guidance in the use of GH at a time when the availability of GH and the promise of effective GH treatment offers what one pediatric endocrinologist calls enthusiastically "an explosion of opportunity."

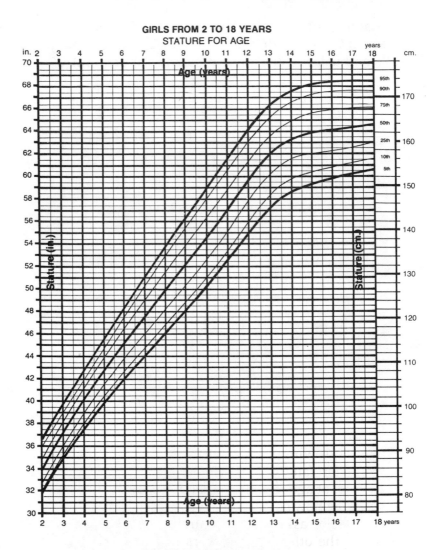

GIRLS FROM 2 TO 18 YEARS
STATURE FOR AGE

NCHS Girl's Growth Chart

Comparing a girl's height with the NCHS norms for girls of the
same age is the most accurate way to evaluate a girl's growth.
Chart distribued by Mead Johnson Nutritionals.

CHAPTER TEN

Finding the Short Kids

The sprinkler is whirling on the lawn; neighborhood children run around. Sarah wants to stand over the sprinkler and feel the water hit against her legs. So does her friend, but there is only room for one. The friend quickly hoists Sarah to her hip and holds her, as mother holds toddler. A natural gesture. What is not natural is that Sarah and her friend are both seven years old; Sarah fits neatly on her friend's hip because she is the size of a four-year-old.

How could this be? Sarah was an average-sized baby, seven pounds five ounces and twenty inches long. Pretty, blond, and lively, Sarah was a happy toddler. She was growing slowly but, with no one to compare her to, her family didn't notice. When she went to preschool at age four, however, her mother, Doris, saw right away how small Sarah was compared to the other children. She asked her pediatrician about it. This doctor, and the other four doctors in the group practice, had written Sarah's height and weight in her record each well visit, but they did not use a growth chart that made comparisons with the norm or with her earlier height. The pediatrician agreed Sarah was small, however, and supposed she had inherited genes for short stature because that is the most common cause of short stature. Doris is 5 feet 6, a taller-than-average mother, and her husband Evan is 5 feet 10, just about the mean height for men, but Doris admitted that her husband had a couple of aunts who were 4 feet 10. That's it, the doctor said, familial short stature; it runs in the family.

Doris tracked her child's growth for three years. "She was dead in the water," says Doris. "She was headed for an adult height way below 5 feet. Sarah herself complained that, when class pictures were taken, the teachers always told her, "Stand on the front row because you are so short." She also complained of having to wear toddler clothes when her friends were wearing school girl fashions.

When Sarah was seven, the family moved across the country. Doris found a new pediatrician and immediately brought up the question of Sarah's height. This doctor saw nothing to get excited about and dutifully recorded the child's growth for three years, again without a chart.

One day Sarah got what appeared to be chicken pox for the second time. Doris, thinking this second outbreak could not be normal, called her pediatrician and found him out of town. She agreed to see the physician on call, an East Indian pediatrician. He took one look at Sarah and, putting aside her chicken pox for the moment, said, "Have you ever had her evaluated for a growth problem?"

For Doris the question was like an alarm, a dash of cold water in the face, a validation of all her concerns. This doctor was the first person who had ever seen what Doris saw, that the child was *abnormally* short.

"No," Doris said, "But how do you get an evaluation for growth?"

The doctor immediately grew cautious. Instead of

answering Doris's question, he asked, "What does your regular doctor say about Sarah's size?"

"He says nothing's wrong."

The new doctor began to pedal backwards, offering no further information.

But Doris now knew there was something that could and should be done. She called on her regular pediatrician when he returned, quoted the question the doctor on call had asked, and demanded a response. The regular pediatrician said he'd have to think about it for a while. Sarah was now ten years old and 4 feet 1 inch, the height of an average seven-year-old.

"Well, if you thought she had a growth problem, what would you do?" Doris asked.

"I'd send her to a specialist—a pediatric endocrinologist," the doctor said.

A pediatric endocrinologist! Doris found one that day in the telephone book, fabricated a referral, and made an appointment.

The specialist recognized within minutes that Sarah could have a growth disorder. She began running tests to find the cause; one was a test for Turner Syndrome, a genetic disorder marked by short stature. It came back positive, although Sarah has no other signs of Turner Syndrome.

When Sarah heard she was going to get GH therapy, she was thrilled. Well, the shots didn't thrill her, and, in fact, she was quite troubled by them for about a week before they became routine. She began treatment with GH in October. Two weeks before Christmas, Sarah and her family went to pick out some shoes she wanted for Christmas that were all the rage in her age group. They were British Knight tennis shoes and they cost $65. Her parents were stunned by the price. Sarah tried on one of the smaller sizes available and they fit.

"I can wear British Knights!" Sarah said to the sales clerk. He shrugged. "You don't understand. I *can* wear British Knights! This is the first time my feet have been big enough to wear what the other kids are wearing. Always before, I had to wear baby shoes." She explained to the clerk that she had to take shots to get big enough for this fashion break-through.

"But $65 for tennis shoes?" Doris looked questioningly at her husband.

"I'd pay $650 just for this experience," he said.

They didn't wait for Christmas. Sarah wore the shoes home that day.

With GH treatment seven days a week, Sarah grew 8 inches in three and a half years, three times the rate she had been growing the year before treatment. At age thirteen she is 4 feet 9 inches. She had a bone age of only eleven years, which means her bone development was two years behind and her growth plates were slow in approaching closure. Her delayed bone age suggests she will have a couple more years of growth and break the 5-feet line that seems like the threshold of normalcy.

When you see the success that Sarah had with GH treatment, you have to wonder why a pediatrician would be so reluctant to refer a short child for evaluation. Perhaps it is because the diagnosis of growth disorder is a relatively new diagnosis. The problem has always been out there, but doctors are not always very aware that it is a medical problem. They are often not familiar with diagnosis and treatment, and, when they are, they may not think the problem justifies the enormous costs of treatment. In addition, parents often seem so preoccupied with their child's height that general practitioners and pediatricians, hearing their complaints, often dismiss them as evidence of societal pressures. Accustomed to over-ambitious parents crying wolf, pediatricians are often reluctant to react. Besides, one pediatric endocrinologist observed, pediatricians in general tend to be short. "If a parent comes in and says, 'If my boy keeps growing at this rate, he will only be 5 feet 5. That's too short. Men in our family are all over 5 feet 10,' the short pediatrician likely will think or say, 'You're the one that has a problem with short stature, not your child.' He will not be interested in pursuing the matter."

Whatever the reason, some growth disorders that could be treated are overlooked.

Take Your Shoes Off and Measure Up

There are tens of thousands of abnormally short children in the U.S. who are candidates for treatment, whether it is GH therapy for GH-deficiency or other appropriate treatment for other growth-retarding disease. But will these children be found?

Kim Frye is director of chapter development for Human Growth Foundation, a national organization that offers support and education to parents of children with growth disorders. "Parents are advocates for their children," says Frye, "and in order to be advocates for their children they need to have education. That's my job. I help the chapters put together educational programs. Not only parents of children on GH therapy are invited but parents of any child with short stature who want information, any parents out there who feel as I did, who are thinking, 'My child is not growing. Where do I go next?' The more education parents receive, the more information they can take to their pediatrician, the more they can insist on explanations until they feel comfortable with their child's treatment or lack of treatment. Then the pediatricians will know they can't just say, '"Don't worry about it."'

Frye believes the majority of children do not have their growth plotted on standard NCHS growth charts. Some children never see a doctor; some doctors do not use the charts. Most parents do not have a way to compare their child's growth to the norms or to their previous growth.

That is why professionals and volunteers associated with the Human Growth Foundation sponsor community and school growth screenings like the one held at Ephesus Elementary school in the small rural town of Bowdon, Georgia. It resembles a typical Health Day activity that might be seen any place in the country. It is different, however, in that the measuring devices and techniques are especially accurate and the visiting health educator has been specially trained in the field of growth.

The gymnasium at Ephesus Elementary is very hot and humid this September day, but the enthusiasm of physical education teacher Susan Dupuy does not seem dampened. Dupuy, who became interested in measuring growth after one of her students was found to be growth hormone deficient, has arranged for the screening led by Pam Kaplan, a health educator from the Atlanta chapter of Human Growth Foundation. Dupuy leads the classes into the gym with seemingly effortless efficiency. They sit quietly on the floor as Kaplan explains that they will be measured very accurately— with bodies straight, shoes off, and bows on top of their hair temporarily removed.

Kaplan calls for a volunteer to go first. An extra tall boy steps up eagerly. First he's weighed. The digital scale reads 42; the boy protests. "That's kilograms," explains Kaplan. Using the metric system facilitates accurate measurement, and it has the added advantage that overweight children—there are more than a few at

Ephesus Elementary—are not embarrassed by the public announcement in more readily understood pounds.

The boy steps over to the stadiometer, a measuring device mounted on the wall that generally allows more accurate measurement than the rule attached to an ordinary scale in a doctor's office. This stadiometer was donated to the school by Human Growth Foundation, courtesy of pharmaceutical company Genentech. Kaplan checks to see that the boy's heels, buttocks, and shoulders are against the wall and his legs straight. She lifts his chin slightly so he's looking straight ahead. Then she swings over the boy's head the measuring arm, determined to be perfectly horizontal by the bubble in the attached level. "You're 147.5 centimeters," she reads from the finely marked rule. For children who may have a growth problem, accuracy to the tenth of a centimeter is important because such a child may grow only a few tenths of a centimeter in a measuring period.

Next Kaplan invites the boy to stand against a life-size growth chart on the wall where his height is compared to the norms for his age. To the older children she explains the percentile marks: the top one marks the 95th percentile, the dark middle line is the 50th percentile line, the bottom line is the 5th percentile. She often adds, "You're growing just fine. She says casually to some children unusually tall or short for their age, "Are your parents tall? Is your mother about as tall as I am?" trying to size up the child's genetic background without seeming intrusive.

Dupuy, who parcels the students out for Kaplan and the school nurse to measure, at the same time conducts PE classes in another part of the gym. As their turns come, small groups of kids, red faced and sweaty, approach the scale, eager for the diversion, eager to please. As their weights are called out—"21 kilograms," "32 kilograms," "28 kilograms"—they ask, "how much is that really?" Kaplan tells them to ask their math teachers to help them convert their measurements to familiar units themselves.

(FYI: To convert kilograms to pounds, multiply the number of kilograms by 2.2. To convert centimeters to inches, multiply the number of centimeters by .3937)

One boy, who measures 172 cm. or almost 5 feet 8 inches, exclaims, "But I can't be five eight! Last year I measured five eleven." Last year, Dupuy points out, the children stood in front of several rulers taped together on the wall and held a book, more or less straight, on their heads. Besides, the boy had been wearing his basketball hightops at the time. From now on, accurate measurement is going to be taken more seriously at Ephesus Elementary.

And so it goes for 180 children, kindergarten through eighth grade. It takes all day. Besides measuring, there is helping kindergarteners get their shoes off and on, getting names spelled right, and—at the end of the day—the all-important task of plotting the figures on the growth charts according to age to the nearest month.

Out of the 180 children, five children fall below the 5th percentile mark on the chart. Notes will be sent to their parents along with a copy of their child's chart informing them that their child is in the lowest percentiles and suggesting they ask their doctor to evaluate this finding. Six children above the 95th percentile were also recorded and notes may be sent to their parents, also.

After his class has been measured, one student stops to talk to Kaplan. Avery is a slender boy with a pleasant childish face, who looks about ten years old. He seems normal in every way—until a glance at his chart reveals he is fourteen years old. Avery's measurement for height is far below the 5th percentile line. His sibling has been measured today near the fortieth percentile.

Is there a health problem here, or just an extreme example of a genetically short child? This is an important question that should be evaluated by a physician. Dupuy has promised to repeat the measurement of every child during the school year to determine growth rate. This measurement will be critical for Avery. If he does not grow significantly between measurements something is definitely wrong. If he does grow a little, the picture is not so clear. Avery's parents may well recognize he is short, but they may not realize how short compared to his agemates.

Abnormally short stature in short families is often overlooked because everyone says, "It's OK, his family is short." Another reason abnormally short stature is often overlooked, says Kaplan, is the phenomenon of juvenilization. Small children are sometimes held back in school by parents to make them appear more like their younger playmates; small children themselves often choose to play with younger children. People often treat small children like younger children, and consequently they tend to take on babyish behavior. They end up seeming like younger children instead of small children of their actual age. "Throw out subjectivity," says Kaplan. "Only accurate measuring and plotting on age-normed charts will identify the short stature child."

Atlanta pediatric endocrinologist Stephen W. Anderson believes screenings like the one at Ephesus School represent one of the best ways to find the children who need attention for growth disorders. "You see a class picture," says Anderson. "And here is Susie at the end of the row, a head shorter than anyone else. Susie never gets to see a pediatric endocrinologist because her family doesn't detect a problem, her physician doesn't detect it as a problem, so she ends up 4 foot 8. That doesn't have to happen. A lot of children are being missed." Anderson remembers the days when many school systems had school nurses who made yearly height and weight measurements which followed a child on his record all the way through school. Children could be compared with their peers from these records. Cutbacks in funding have eliminated this approach in most places. Anderson hopes volunteer efforts will begin to meet this need.

Growth screenings by the Human Growth Foundation have flagged children with short stature, who, upon examination, were found to have serious problems such as brain tumors, Turner's Syndrome, and thyroid deficiency. "Failure to grow is often the first sign of some underlying disease," says Kaplan.

One concern is that children who are flagged by a growth screening get a good evaluation by their doctors or at a health clinic. Besides conducting growth screenings, Kaplan goes to pediatricians' offices and talks to staffs about the need for frequent and accurate growth measurements and plots on standard growth charts. Beyond the first grade physical, parents often do not take their children for wellness check-ups every two years as is commonly recommended by pediatricians. Kaplan urges measurements be plotted on a growth chart at every visit, sick or well, so there will be a detailed record of growth over time.

"My, How You've Grown! When I Last Saw You, You Were This High!"

In normal children, skeletal growth does not occur evenly over childhood, of course. A child's greatest growth rate occurs before birth. The size of a baby at birth has more to do with the mother's system than the baby's. Shortly after birth, the baby's own characteristics take over. A baby will usually reach his genetically determined growth channel by age two or three years of age and stay in it till puberty or beyond.

Growth is very rapid at first; an average baby will grow about 25 cm. (almost ten inches) the first year of life. In the second year, a baby will typically grow another 10 to 15 cm. (about 4 to 6 inches), and after that it's all downhill. Growth rate levels off to a steady rate of about 5 to 6 cm. (about 2 to 2.4 inches) per year until the pubertal growth spurt of 8 to 10 cm. (about 3 to 4 inches) per year. After this spurt, growth tapers off till the growth plates fuse at about age 16 for girls and 18 for boys.

The growth spurt at puberty begins on the average a year or two earlier in girls (about age 11) than in boys (about age 13) and varies widely within each group. Anyone who has ever chaperoned a junior high school dance knows that the timing of this event for both girls and boys varies dramatically—sometimes with comic, sometimes with painful effect. After puberty, growth will taper off until adult height is soon reached and the growth plates close.

Growth hormone levels in the blood after infancy follow a similar pattern as growth rate, with the biggest spurt occurring at puberty. Beyond the general similarity of pattern, GH levels in normal children do not correlate with height. Normal tall children, for example, have not been found to secrete spontaneously more GH on the average than normal shorter children. They may instead have a greater sensitivity to GH. At puberty, kids experience more frequent GH surges during the day and bigger surges at night, especially the boys. Girls are less consistent with most of their increase observed in the waking hours. Of course, girls do not have as far to grow.

How Short Is Too Short?

"It seems to me my child is too short."

"When is my child going to grow?"

"But his friends are so much taller!"

"I do hope she'll be taller than I am."

Parents often express these concerns about their children's stature. Not infrequently children themselves complain.

"I can imagine how painful it must be to be a short child," says one 6-feet-3-inch child psychiatrist, "only because I can remember the pleasure I felt when people constantly admired my above-average height when I was a child. The short child's feelings of lack of approval must be equally keen."

The advantages of height are well documented; studies show that taller adults make more money and achieve more leadership roles than their shorter peers. Children of every size often boast that they intend to grow to a certain height, to the stature of an ideal athlete or a model or dancer, as if wishing could make them grow. Most kids adjust well to reality if they do not reach their goal; some do not.

In any case, half of all children are below average in height by definition and, statistically speaking, every population is expected to have a few extreme values that are nonetheless normal.

Short stature, as a disorder, is defined by Emory University's John S. Parks as "a height below the range appropriate for a child or adolescent's age, gender, and genetic background." Using NCHS (National Center for Health Statistics) growth charts, like the girls' chart at the beginning of this chapter, Parks plots measurements to address the following questions:

a. How tall is the child compared to other children the same age? Plot the child's height for his age and estimate the height percentile. Is the child in the 50th or the 5th percentile of height for age? If below the 5th, then calculate how far below.

b. How tall is the child compared to the parents? Plot the parents' heights in the percentile channels far to the right. (When possible, measure the parent because adults tend to inflate their height by 1 1/2 inches on the average!) Add 5 inches to put a mother on a male child's chart or subtract 5 inches to put a father on a female child's chart. This adjustment reflects the mean difference in adult heights between men and women. Estimate the mid point between the parents' height percentiles and compare this with the child's height percentile.

c. How did the child arrive at his/her current height? Plot past measurements to distinguish between slow but steady growth and growth arrest.

Children usually enter their genetically determined growth channels between the ages of two and three years. With good health and adequate nutrition, they stay in these channels until puberty. Women mature earlier than men and experience two fewer years of childhood growth at a rate of about 2 1/2 inches per year, accounting for the 5-inch difference in adult height. Early maturers of either sex tend to wind up relatively short, while late maturers are relatively tall. In any case, most short or tall children are growing normally for their genetic backgrounds.

The following patterns, Parks says, should be considered abnormal and demand investigation:

a. Height below the 1st percentile. There is a reasonable chance of detecting a disease process at this extreme degree of short stature. There is a much lower probability of a treatable disease process in children between the 5th and 1st percentiles.

b. Height more than three channels below the midparental channel. For example, if both parents are in the 90th percentile for height, there is a reasonable chance that their son in the 10th percentile is not meeting his genetic potential for growth.

c. Crossing of two or more channels after two years of age. The large baby of short parents will usually grow at a "sub-normal" rate in infancy while seeking his genetically determined growth channel. After two years of age, however, deviations of this magnitude usually indicate a disease process.

Children whose short stature meets these criteria for abnormality should be thoroughly evaluated. For example, the physician will determine whether the child's weight for his height suggests a particular disorder. A measurement of head circumference and length of limbs and trunk will determine proportionality.

The physician will also want to determine whether the child's pubertal stage is appropriate for his/her chronological age. Parks notes, for example, that in genetic short stature, pubertal development is on time.

These children are short for age, but they do not look young for age. Absence of age-appropriate pubertal development in a girl, together with somes other mild features may reflect Turner Syndrome. Children with hypopituitarism or with constitutional delay of growth tend to look young for age during childhood and fail to enter puberty at a normal age. Hypothyroidism, on the other hand, may be present with premature puberty without an appropriate pubertal growth spurt.

Many of the disorders responsible for growth impairment will be obvious during a careful history and physical examination, says Parks. Then laboratory studies will be necessary to confirm a clinical hypothesis. A great many disorders can be verified by a routine urinalysis and blood work-up. More specialized studies like a thyroid function study may also be necessary.

When other more common disorders are ruled out, testing for GH production becomes appropriate.

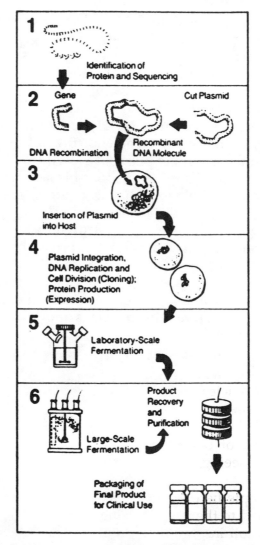

Recombinant DNA Product Development

The gene of interest is identified and isolated (steps 1 and 2) and then cloned into a microorganism or host cell (steps 3 and 4). The recombinant protein is produced and purified for clinical use (steps 5 and 6). *Reprinted with permission of Genentech.*

From Clone to Clinic: The Drug Companies

S tainless steel tanks shoot up like skyscrapers into a network of pipes. Attendants rustle in and out in paper moonsuits. They take readings, adjust knobs, make notes.

Inside the tanks a mysterious and important process is going on that must be attended with ritualistic motions as a queen bee's nest must be attended by worker bees or an oracle must be guarded by her priestesses. A high-tech laboratory, a shrine to DNA, a surreal incubator.

"It's sort of like making beer," says a Genentech employee, seeing nothing either holy or surreal about it.

The people here at Genentech's plant have become accustomed to the miracle being performed by the Escherichia coli inside the tanks as a broth of pampered bacteria churns out biosynthetic growth hormone for the waiting market.

Escherichia coli, called e. coli for short, is a much maligned bacterium normally found in the intestinal tract of humans and other mammals. While e. coli in water can cause urinary infections, in its proper place, it is more helpful than harmful. As an inhabitant of the digestive tract, its presence in river water or a well is a mark of human waste pollution.

But, in its proper place, domesticated, the little microbe can be induced to do some very useful things. Through genetic engineering, specifically, recombinant DNA technology, the human gene for GH is inserted into a DNA molecule of the bacteria, which is then cloned. These engineered e. coli are thus "tricked" into producing growth hormone. In commercial production, the bacteria are kept in tanks, dark and warm inside, like the finest intestines they could want, well fed as if by a host both gourmet and gourmand. There they can gurgle and ferment and produce to their hearts' content. Their product is periodically siphoned off to undergo purifying processes.

After the biosynthetic GH is purified, it will be sealed in sturdy little bottles. Each bottle of clear GH extract, containing enough GH for about three injections, will be packed with a slightly taller bottle of bacteriostatic water preserved with benzyl alcohol that must be mixed with the GH for injection. The GH must be refrigerated to keep it inactive so its large molecules won't break down into smaller molecules of unknown substances.

And all the notes taken about its generation and distribution will be scrutinized by the quality control monitors, by the FDA, by the auditors. GH is a very closely tracked substance.

Genentech is not the only company in the world that makes GH, nor even the only company in the country. But Genentech was the first company allowed by the FDA to market the drug in the U.S. The journey from the biochemistry lab at the University of California

CHAPTER ELEVEN

where C.H. Li synthesized the GH molecule to the mass production of the substance at commercial levels was a long and expensive one. Any company making this journey would have to believe the results would ultimately be profitable.

The U.S. government offers incentives to companies like Genentech to research and develop a new drug that relatively few people will ever buy by awarding "orphan drug" status to the drug. The 1983 Orphan Drug Act was enacted by Congress (Public Law 97-414) to encourage development, testing, and production of drugs that are effective and safe for the treatment of rare diseases. These drugs are deemed unlikely to be profitable for a drug company to develop without special allowances. Such drugs were called "orphan" drugs because, presumably, nobody wants to "raise" them. Orphan drug status can be given only to a drug likely to be appropriate for fewer than 200,000 people in the U.S. at any one time.

The law offers the designated pharmaceutical company tax credits, fewer regulatory barriers, and—best of all—exclusivity in the market. For seven years from the award of this status, no other drug company is allowed to market the same drug. About 350 drugs have been given orphan status since the law was passed, far more than were developed under the longer period prior to 1983 when the federal government and other institutions were funding research and development without protecting the individual drug market. Genentech's GH was one of the first pharmaceutical products to achieve the designation of orphan drug.

Genentech's synthetic version of GH was called *somatrem* by the scientific community to distinguish it from *somatotropin,* the GH naturally produced by the human pituitary. Genentech's version was also called *met-GH* to indicate that it was not an exact copy of natural GH. With a molecular weight of 192, it had an extra amino acid, methionine, not present in the pituitary product. The extra methionine particle was an artifact of the particular method of producing GH, but the resultant hormone had the same properties as pituitary GH. European companies also produced somatrem or met-GH by similar methods. Genentech began to market its product under the brand-name Protropin (R).

Protropin was a huge success clinically—and at the bank. By 1988 yearly sales of Protropin came to over $100 million, pushing the little biotech research company that developed it into the heady world of drug manufacturers. It is not known what the research and development of the hormone cost Genentech, but the average cost of developing a new drug has been estimated at $200 million spread over a twelve year period. Pricing of the orphan product is not exactly arbitrary, but it is certainly an arcane process not overseen by the government. Many questions figure in the decision: Should the price reflect expected sales for the remainder of the seven year "orphan" period? For a longer period? For a shorter period? Should the price cover costs of the research and development specifically for that product or should they cover their fair share of corporate overhead? Should the price be set to carry the company through some of its less successful ventures? Or should it be what the market will bear? No matter what price a company picks, there are likely to be accusations that the latter criteria was the guiding one.

Two years after Genentech put Protropin on the market, Indianapolis-based Eli Lilly and Company requested and obtained orphan drug status for its biosynthetic GH product designed to treat the same population. This designation appeared to violate the exclusivity Genentech had been enjoying for Protropin. Technically, however, the FDA concluded, it did not, and Genentech failed to win a restraining order to block distribution of the Lilly product. Lilly's GH was slightly different in molecular structure. Vive la difference! Unlike Protropin, Lilly's product, called somatropin and marketed under the brand name Humatrope (R), was an exact copy of human growth hormone with the same 191 amino acids as the real thing— "authentic" recombinant growth hormone, as Lilly says. The difference between Genentech's Protropin and Lilly's Humatrope was, at the time, considered important.

The early batches of Protropin had been associated with a high level of antibodies in the children treated with it. Antibodies, products of the immune system, are nature's weapons against unwanted outside substances. Antibodies attack the intruders, bind with them, and clear them from the system. Antibodies to exogenous GH could potentially make GH useless. Although pituitary GH had also provoked antibodies at about the same level, the antibodies to Protropin were supposed by many to be reacting to the extra amino acid, methionine, which it recognized as foreign. Although very few patients failed to grow with Protropin, the antibodies were worrisome and a more authentic version of biosynthetic GH seemed desirable. Lilly got the go-ahead to produce methionyl-free GH under the Orphan Law.

In the meantime, new methods of extracting GH from its bacterial host cleared up a portion of Protropin's antibody formation which was determined to be in response to a protein contaminant from the e. coli rather than the methionine residue. The incidence of formation of antibodies to GH itself remains higher for Protropin (30%) than for Humatrope (2%), but cases of failure to grow with Protropin (as for Humatrope) have been so few as to be insignificant. Those antibodies were non-binding and so did not interfere with the function of GH, Genentech explains. Lilly continues to point out the authenticity of Humatrope and its low incidence of associated antibodies.

So the two companies split the market that was once categorized as unprofitable for even one company. In 1990 Genentech had 75% of the $200 million U.S. market. While most people choosing GH for the first time might be expected to choose the "authentic" GH over the slightly inexact version, doctors, unconcerned with the difference between the products, prescribe Protropin three times more often than Humatrope perhaps because Protropin came out first, performed well, and doctors see no reason to change. Also figuring heavily in the sales preference are Genentech's greater number of company representatives assigned to GH and higher profile publicity. For Genentech, with a predicted 1991 total sales figure of $500 million, the Protropin sales are a really big deal. Lilly, by contrast, as a company with a predicted $6 billion in 1991 total sales, does not rely so heavily on Humatrope and markets it less aggressively. Even so, Lilly's $40 to $50 million chunk of the U.S. market along with additional sales worldwide are nothing to sniff at.

In 1990 a congressional hearing was held to discuss the large profits some drug companies were making on certain orphan drugs. GH was one of three drugs discussed. The question was posed whether orphan drugs which had developed a much larger market than predicted should have their orphan status shortened. As far as GH was concerned, it was almost too late to ask.

In 1992 the orphan drug market protection period lapses for Genentech's product; in 1994 Lilly's exclusivity expires. Any company may then jump into the GH market and several are poised for the plunge. But the legal area of production rights are much more complex than they appear at first glance, and every new wrinkle in the technology has its own patent. The companies share and lease and argue over them. Highly paid patent attorneys account for a big chunk of the drug company outlay. Over the years Genentech has been sued by another pharmaceutical company, Hoffman-LaRoche, and even by the C.H. Li's old outfit, the Hormone Research Foundation of University of California in San Francisco, over patent rights to certain processes of GH synthesis; Genentech in turn has sued the FDA over its criteria for awarding Orphan Drug status based on the drug's structure rather than its process of synthesis.

When the dust settles, the new competition, which may involve six or seven companies, will undoubtedly drive down consumer costs of GH somewhat. One physician, formerly associated with Olympic drug testing, guessed the price could go as low as $10 to $20 a month, a figure which would enormously relieve parents of GH-deficient children, who now pay about $1,500 a month, but would also favor the illicit distribution of GH. Most experts expect a more modest drop in price. In any case, the drug companies can expect the market for GH to expand one way or another as prices ease.

Once a drug is approved for use in one medical situation, there is no legal prohibition against its use for other "off-label" situations at the physician's discretion. Barry Werth in his *New York Times Magazine* article describes a strategy that leads from a federally guaranteed monopoly on a drug labeled for use for a rare disorder to an enormous off-label market. "The big money with an increasing number of drugs is not with those few indications covered by the FDA label but with those many, many more that aren't. Indeed, a good part of the game in drug marketing is now to find the narrowest indications possible for drugs that are likely to be block-busters later on."

Werth continues, "The success of Genentech's hand-holding of doctors and patients, its exploiting of gaps in knowledge, its leveraging of enormously favorable Federal regulations and its blurring of the line between sickness and health, all can be measured most strikingly in Protropin's sales." The 1990 sales of $157 million of Protropin, up 40% over 1988 belies the GH status as a drug that nobody wanted. The orphan, it seems, was always expected to be the golden goose.

The drug companies, however, did not invent the idea of remedying shortness as if it were a disease, as Werth implies. In his *New York Times Magazine* article, he says that the Oriti family was getting human pituitary GH for Marco even before the synthetic product was available from Genentech. In the 1940s, extra short guys went to a local gym and swung from ropes in hopes of stretching their vertebrae out a half inch so they could get into the Marines. Long before Protropin, people noticed the "tall" in "tall, dark, and handsome" and the higher salaries, voter preference, and sports success of the tall. The idea of wanting to be tall may be on the rise, but it has always been there—to be exploited perhaps, but not to be invented. Moreover, the distinction of creating a disease is one the medical world makes; it's not one the consumer cares about. For decades, people have paid for orthodontia for buckteeth, for example; no one asked, wait a minute, are buckteeth a disease? No one pondered, "My father has buckteeth, too; I guess it's inherited, so, knowing that,

I am content with being called 'Rabbit' by the kids at school."

GH treatment is more risky, more burdensome, and less certain of outcome than orthodontia, and so is ethically inadvisable except for carefully chosen candidates, but the desire for treatment of short stature has apparently been there waiting for at least as long as the drug companies have been researching a remedy. Adult desire for more muscle and less fat, though not new, has been increasing independently from drug-company-supported explorations.

Drug companies marketing GH in the U.S. are not allowed to label or advertise the drug for any use other than that which the FDA has approved. In addition, Dr. David Kessler, the FDA commissioner, in 1991 announced his intention of cracking down on drug companies and perhaps doctors that privately promote a drug for a use not listed on the agency label. But GH manufacturers have from the beginning carefully tracked GH distribution to deter off-label use, the drug companies say, while supporting many approved experimental studies such as those whose results have been summarized in this book.

In 1985, when Protropin was approved for marketing, Genentech sought a distribution system that had more controls than the ordinary network of pharmaceutical wholesalers and drugstores but fewer controls than is required for narcotics. Genentech set up a distribution system through home health care companies. Home health care companies, which provide drug therapy, generally long term, for homebound patients, are ideally suited for the distribution of GH because they keep good records. Genentech's distribution has the benefits of Caremark's security, patient files, and quality control auditing. Eighty % of Genentech's sales are through Caremark Homecare and its affiliated regional spin-off companies.

The remaining 20% of Protropin sales are direct sales to the federal government for military families or to HMOs and hospitals whose physicians are limited and subject to organizational scrutiny. Before any shipment of Protropin is made to a new account, Genentech confirms that the prescription is written by a pediatric endocrinologist and only for approved use. If an order comes in from a general practioner or other specialist, Genentech asks for a referral to a pediatric endocrinologist. When Eli Lilly's Humatrope was approved for sale, Lilly opted for a similar system, using New England Critical Care as its main distributor.

The National Cooperative Growth Study (NCGS) is an additional resource for tracking Protropin's use. More than 80 percent of children treated with the drug have participated in this Genentech-sponsored study. Among the most comprehensive post-marketing surveillance studies ever undertaken, the NCGS has enrolled more than 11,000 children since its inception in 1985. Only children with growth disorders may participate in the study and their use of Protropin is regularly monitored until treatment is discontinued.

And as much as we would like to separate the attainment of normal stature from issues of dollars and cents, the two are entwined. All the activity behind the thousands of heart warming stories like Michael's, Danielle's, and Brent's is, after all, an industry, a growing industry, and any complete story of GH must include a look at the business of growth.

CHAPTER TWELVE

GH and Adults: Antidote to Aging, Boon to Fertility and Healing?

When Walter reached an adult height of 5 feet 4 inches and his doctor told him his growth plates had closed and that's all the height that could be squeezed out of his growth hormone therapy, he felt a pang of disappointment and then a sudden relief that it was all over. No more needles, no more alcohol and swabs, no more dragging around an ice chest on every trip. Free.

Walter had no thought that now he would be a GH-deficient adult. It did not cross his mind that GH was good for anything more than producing those precious inches. It's just as well. His doctor would not have prescribed more GH for him even if he'd been willing; certainly his family would not want to pay for it. They had been counting the days until that burden was off their backs.

But GH does play a role in normal adult life and lack of it has some effect on life even after skeletal growth stops. "Growth hormone," says Daniel Rudman, "has a powerful effect on body composition and on the functions of most organs except the nervous system." In normal adults, GH secretion, although lower than at its peak during puberty, finds a level that may go on unchanged for decades. This normal level of GH causes cell proliferation and repair of muscles, bones, and skin. The right amount of circulating GH keeps the liver and kidney at an optimum size and level of function. GH also has a role in the growth of lymphoid tissue including thymus, lymph nodes, spleen and bone marrow, all of which are integral to the immune system. GH maintains fluid levels. It keeps fat in check. Not only does GH keep fat in a better proportion to muscle, but GH keeps extra fat in the healthier "pear" distribution rather than "apple" distribution. Or to put it more earthily, GH favors "butt over gut." A distribution of relatively greater hip and thigh fat has been found to be associated with fewer health threats like heart attacks and diabetes than extra weight carried higher on the belly and midriff.

Without GH

Without GH, the cell proliferation of otherwise normal adults declines two- to ten-fold, and they do not thrive as well as their contemporaries with a full measure of the hormone.

Indeed, even young GH-deficient adults tend to be overweight with a lower than normal lean body mass. To give an idea of the magnitude of the difference, the distribution of muscle and fat in the thigh of GH-deficient adult subjects, studied by Swedish doctor Bengt-Ake Bengtsson, was 65% muscle and 35% fat, while the ratio of muscle to fat in the thigh of normal adults is 85% to 15%. Bengtsson, like Rudman, found that a few months' treatment with GH completely or partially normalized the fat-to-muscle proportion in these GH-deficient adults.

There is also evidence, not yet conclusive, that GH-deficiency may reduce muscular strength along with muscle mass. A research team headed by Ross Cuneo studied 24 adults who had suffered a GH deficiency for a year or more. These patients, who were matched with normal controls of similar age, size, and activity level, also had less strength in their quadriceps (the large muscle on the front of the thigh). In some subjects, strength was even less than might be expected from their reduced muscle mass. At Stanford University, Raymond Hintz has done a study of GH, the GH-dependent growth factor Sm-C/IGF-I, and grip strength of aging men and women. Preliminary results showed a correlation between grip strength and Sm-C/IGF-I levels. Those who were low in the GH-dependent growth factor didn't have as strong a grip.

Moreover, patients with GH deficiency often complain of lethargy, according to Cuneo, who speculates that muscles lacking normal mass may fatigue more easily. Another possibility, says Cuneo is that a shortage of GH may mean a change in the muscles' storage or use of glucose, sugar used as an energy source. After all, Sm-C/IGF-I is partially responsible for stimulating transport of glucose into skeletal muscle. Without glucose, muscles don't work, and you don't work.

It has also been observed that a deficiency of GH is often accompanied by a decline in growth of natural killer cells, those warriors of the immune system which attack invaders such as tumor cells.

In addition, there is evidence that GH-deficient individuals, whether children or adults, are "psychologically compromised." Psychological adjustment is tough to measure, but some researchers have tried.

Two groups of researchers doing follow-up studies of patients treated for GH-deficiency in childhood found that, as GH-deficient adults, they were more likely than their peers to be single and unemployed. Some of these GH-deficient individuals are no doubt abnormally small, but small stature in general has not been found to be an impediment to marriage and employment.

For those of you who may be offended that single-hood—or unemployment, for that matter—is psychologically "compromising", other researchers have used criteria you might prefer. British researchers G.A. McGauley and colleagues of St. Thomas Hospital in London and University Hospital in Zurich used three different quality-of-life assessments to test 24 adults who met strict criteria for GH-deficiency. The tests showed lower scores for the GH-deficient than for the normal controls matched for age, gender, ethnic origin, socio-economic level, and area of residence. After six months of treatment with GH, the GH-deficient subjects experienced less perceived illness and improvements in their perception of energy level and mood than the control group which had received placebos.

Adults who have lost pituitary function from radiation treatment, surgery, or disease, have their thyroid, adrenal, and gonadal hormones routinely replaced as appropriate, but growth hormone, considered unessential, is generally not replenished. The value of adult GH is acknowledged but not considered critical—or proven safe—or worth the price—by many physicians and the FDA.

"Our present knowledge," said J. Sandahl Christiansen and colleagues at Danish research centers in 1990, "strongly supports the concept that GH is not only important for skeletal growth and tissue development in childhood and adolescence, but is also of critical importance for the maintenance of these structures during adult life. This, together with the other beneficial effects of GH replacement reported..., brings us the conclusion that lifelong GH replacement in GH-deficient patients, whether GH deficient since childhood or with acquired GH deficiency in adult life, should be considered. Further long-term studies are needed in order to finally establish the potential benefits of GH replacement therapy which then, and only then, will have to be compared to the costs of such treatment."

Most Likely to Be Growth Hormone Deficient: The Elderly

Because of the ebb and flow of birthrate in this century and because of rising life expectancies, the elderly today make up an increasing proportion of our population. The health and well being of the elderly is critical to all of us. They are, however, weaker, flabbier, paunchier, more stooped, more prone to bone fractures and dental breakdown, and less resistant to disease than their younger counterparts. These characteristics are the immutable results of age itself. Or are they? Is there not some concrete, observable process that brings on the symptoms of aging? Something measurable, reachable, even changeable?

Perhaps. The link between aging and growth hormone level is certainly a strong one. "After about age 50," says Rudman, "the secretion of growth hormone (GH) gradually declines and ultimately stops in many individuals. About half our citizens over age 65, therefore, are partially or totally deficient in GH. The hypothesis arises, therefore, that several of the geriatric changes in structure and function result at least in part from GH deficiency."

Here are the changes that come with age, noted by

Rudman and others. Compare these changes with the alterations attributed to GH-deficiency:

In healthy youth, says Rudman, about 10% of the body weight is bone, 30% is muscle, and 20% is fat tissue. After about age 50, these ratios change progressively. At age 75, a typical composition is 8% bone, 15% muscle, and 40% fat, that is, 20% less bone, half the muscle, and twice the fat. Besides having twice the fat, the fat moves around, going to gut.

Although women generally have more fat than men, both men and women show variations of the same pattern of change. A study reported by Margaret Flynn and collegues at the University of Washington-Columbia, followed 564 males and 61 females for 18 years (1969-1987). Lean body mass, roughly the same as muscle mass, was calculated for all subjects, mostly members of the faculty at the university, ranging from 28 to 60 years of age. Each subject after age 40 showed some loss of lean body mass even though the group's average weight was relatively stable. Men experienced gradual loss of lean with the most rapid decrease between ages 41 and 60. Women, although they had a higher proportion of fat at every age than men, tended to keep what muscle they had longer; their rapid loss of muscle occurred in the decade after age 60. Sorry to say, in their pattern of change, those men and women who had been regularly running, jogging, or cycling were not significantly different from those who were less active.

Muscles not only make up a smaller proportion of the body with advancing age, muscle strength also falls. For example, muscle strength of ten muscle groups of 75-year-old men is only 40% to 60% as great as in 35-year-old men, reports Rudman.

Changes in bone mass with age are particularly serious. Bone is constantly being "remodeled" by continuing *formation*, i.e., building up, and *resorption*, i.e., the process by which the calcium-building blocks of bone are torn down and reabsorbed into the blood. The formation of bone is greater than the tearing down through about age 30 and bone mass increases; after that the tearing down exceeds the building up, explains Rudman. Men lose bone mass gradually while women maintain nearly the same level until the decade between ages 50 and 60. Rapid loss of bone mass is called *osteoporosis*. The results of this condition are that older people often suffer fractures of the hip and limbs, which leave them bedridden. Compressions of the spinal column as vertebrae collapse cripples some elderly people and causes others to stoop. Also, loss of bone mass in the jaws accounts to some extent for loss of teeth in the elderly.

And what's the one organ most readily associated with advancing age? Skin. Wrinkles and lines. Furrows, crinkles, and crows' feet. Few serious investigators have been tempted to count wrinkles or record their depth. They have, however, been willing to measure skin thickness and the amount of collagen, a protein necessary to the structure of skin. British investigators Sam Shuster and colleagues in 1975 set about making measurements to be used as a standard normal reference in future studies and when observing skin in disease. The subjects were 74 males and 80 women aged 15 to 93. They found that men had more collagen than women at any age and that collagen in both declined directly with age, about 1% per year throughout adult life. The thickness of skin, which is related but not identical to collagen, told a slightly different story. Males experienced a gradual thinning of skin with advancing age; women's skin thickness remained constant until age fifty, after which it decreased. In adult skin, the clinical features of aging are closely related to the total collagen content.

Other less visible organs are also affected by age. The kidneys decrease in size about 30% between the ages of 30 and 75. Along with reduction in size there is about a 50% decrease in blood flow and filtering capability. There is diminished ability to conserve and excrete substances (salt, for example) as needed. Age affects the kidneys' ability to process vitamin D, which, among other things, regulates calcium needed to build up bone. Liver size and blood flow are reduced by an average of 30% between ages 30 and 75. Older people are, therefore, less able to clear drugs from their systems. The spleen loses about 50% of its mass, and several immune responses are impaired.

When writers refer metaphorically to "a dried-up" old person, they may be more literally accurate than they think. With age, total body water decreases. Sweating is also reduced and the body's cooling system becomes less efficient.

So there it is: Aging and GH-deficiency at any age are associated with the same set of changes, from skin to bones, tit for tat. Similarly, GH-therapy and even GH excess (with all its dangers) move the body in the opposite direction. Because of the similarity between the symptoms of GH-deficiency and the symptoms of old age, it is not going out on a limb to say that a decrease in GH in the elderly makes some contribution to the general decline in old age. The following table adapted from one in an 1985 article by Rudman published in the *Journal of the American Geriatric Society* illustrates the parallels between aging and GH level.

Summary of Structure/Function Changes Attributed to Age, Growth Hormone Deficiency and Excess

Change:	with age	GH deficiency	GH excess
Function			
Muscle mass	↓	↓	↑
Muscle strength	↓	?	?
Bone mass	↓	↓	↑
Bone density	↓	↓	→
Lower jaw bone size	↓	↓	↑
Kidney size	↓	↓	↑
Kidney blood flow	↓	↓	↑
Glomerular filtration rate	↓	↓	→
Calcium absorption	↓	?	?
Liver size	↓	↓	↑
BSP clearance	↓	?	?
Fat mass	↑	↑	↓
Spleen size	↓	↓	↑

GH = growth hormone; Glomerular filtration rate is a measure of kidney function; BSP clearance = bromsuphthalein clearance, a measure of liver function; ↓ = decrease; ↑ = increase; → = remains the same; ? = unknown.

(Adapted from Rudman, D.: Growth Hormone, Body Composition, and Aging. *Journal of the American Geriatrics Society*, Nov. 1987, pp. 800-807. (Used with permission of the Journal of the American Geriatric Society)

Rudman's study of GH with elderly men suggests that replacement GH might be appropriate for those elderly individuals whose GH is below normal. However, while more than one of Rudman's subjects has expressed the wish to be back on GH treatment, Rudman himself does not suggest that GH should be in long term general use for the elderly. There have been, in adult studies, some side effects which, though not worrisome under the scrutiny and control of the researchers, could be dangerous in less well-monitored situations. And the concurrence between age-related changes and disorders related to GH-deficiency does not automatically mean GH treatment would solve the problems.

Another deterrent to long term use of GH replacement therapy where levels of the hormone fall below normal is that there is uncertainty about the normal adult level of GH. The fact that half of all individuals over 65 may stop secreting GH and the other half keep on secreting GH makes us question which state is normal. For whom, if anyone, would GH replacement therapy constitute an overdose?

Short term use of GH to build up a person seems more likely than long term use to be a practical reality in the near future. Ike, for example, a frail 78-year-old man cannot feed himself. Nursing home attendants bring his meals three times a day. They set the trays down in front of him and go on to other patients. When—and if—they have time, they may come back and feed him, slow mouthful, by slow mouthful. Chances are they will give up before he has had his fill. Naturally, Ike is getting weaker. He is not ready for a feeding tube; he can chew and swallow. All he needs is a boost to his hand, wrist, and arm muscles and he could get the food to his own mouth at his own pace. Is this a job for GH? Some say an exercise program would do as much or more for Ike than GH treatment would. Perhaps so. And perhaps exercise and GH therapy together would be a definitive boost that would put Ike back in the ranks of the self-feeding.

Especially Women

You probably couldn't help noticing in the previous pages the repetition of this thought: "Men lose..... (bone mass, muscle tissue, skin thickness)...gradually, while women maintain the same levels until after age 50 when there is a rapid decline." When you realize that the age mentioned is about the age of menopause, the cessation of estrogen secretion in women, you might begin to think the two events are connected. And you would be right. Estrogen deficiency and GH deficiency are linked, as we have noted before in the section on Turner's Syndrome.

Young women secrete about 50% more GH than young men. If this surprises you because you see that women grow less tall than men, remember that puberty comes a couple years sooner for women and they have two fewer years to grow.

Early studies showed that at about age 30 a gradual decline in GH production often begins, and at some point some people stop making it altogether. It seemed that GH secretion just slips away like other signs of youth. But some of these studies used men as subjects and some used both men and women. Some studies used fat and skinny people without taking into account the fact that obesity itself seems to be an inhibitor of GH secretion. These variables made clarifying patterns of GH loss difficult.

In the late 1980s some researchers at the University of Virginia, including K.Y. Ho and Michael Thorner, decided to untangle some of these factors to get a clearer picture of when, how much, and for whom GH declines. They hitched IVs up to 36 normal adult subjects for a solid day and night. The researchers told the subjects what to eat and when to sleep while a 24-hour profile of their GH secretion was recorded.

Then Ho, Thorner, and company analyzed the data. They looked at total GH, amplitudes of peak production, age, sex, weight, and levels of estradiol (one of the most active estrogens) and testosterone in *both men and women* (see charts on facing page).

The subjects fell into one of two age groups: younger (18 to 30 years old) and older (56 to 71 years old). As expected, the young women had more GH than the young men, and the older subjects, both women and men, had less GH than the younger subjects. Also, as expected, the women's decline had been very sharp while the men's was only slight so that the older women ended up with the same or less GH than the older men. It had been known that women's GH takes a plunge right about the time of menopause. It certainly seemed as if the GH picture to some extent mirrored the estrogen picture in women. But to what extent? And what about men?

That's the beauty of the study by Ho, Thorner et al. The researchers measured the sex steroid concentrations of all the subjects: Both men and women had measurable estradiol (estrogen) levels; the young women had about twice as much of the so-called female hormone as the men. Similarly, the young men and young women both had measurable testosterone, but the young men had about 20 times as much of the so-called male hormone as the women. When the researchers looked at how testosterone and GH related (holding other variables constant), they came up empty handed. But when they looked at estradiol levels, they found that release of GH correlates very clearly with estradiol. The researchers concluded that sex and age have both independent and interrelated effects on GH

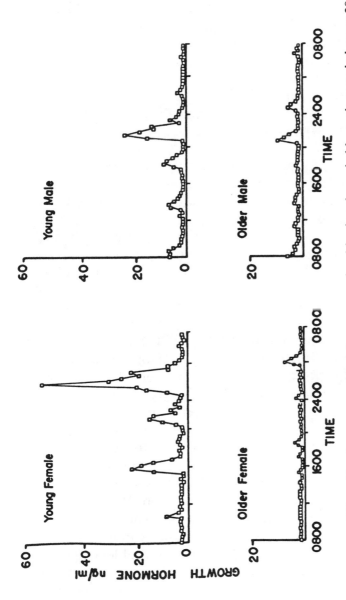

Representative GH profiles from a young female, young male, older female, and older male sampled every 20 minutes for 24 hours. Pulses were categorized as large (L) or small (S) depending on whether the rise was greater or less than three times the threshold criterion for a pulse. *From Ho K.Y., Evans W.S., Blizzard R.M., Veldhuis J.D., Merriam G.R., Samojlik E., Furlanetto R., Rogol A.D., Kaiser D.L., and Thorner M.O. Used with permission of The Endocrine Society from "Effects of Sex and Age on the 24-Hour Profile of Growth Hormone Secretion in Man," Journal of Clinical Endocrinology and Metabolism, 1987; vol. 64, pp. 51-57.*

secretion which can be largely accounted for by corresponding variations in endogenous estradiol levels. Indeed, by removing the variability due to free estradiol, the effects of sex and age on GH secretion are no longer significant, the researchers conclude.

Now it all makes sense. Young women have more estrogen than men and they have more growth hormone. Similarly, young women taking oral contraceptives high in estrogen have greater GH production than other women their age not on the pill. When women reach menopause, their estrogen level falls down and GH comes tumbling after. Men lose their share of estrogen, too, only its not such a big deal for them because the loss is gradual and they only had half as much to begin with. So it could be that weakened bones, shifts of flesh from the muscle to the fat side, thinning skin, and all that other aging stuff are just as much a result of GH loss as of estrogen loss or some other aspect of aging.

So where does that possibility lead? Some investigators, like Rudman, immediately thought of injecting GH to help turn back some of the changes of aging. But the first question that leaps to every older woman's mind is this: if GH decline is related to estrogen levels, will estrogen replacement after menopause bring back more youthful levels of GH?

Estrogen Replacement and GH

Yes, there is enough evidence that exogenous estrogen will raise GH levels that quite a bit of research is being done on that very matter. "The positive effect of estrogens on pulsatile GH secretion has important implications," says Ho, Thorner, et al., citing the benefits of adequate GH on protein synthesis, muscle mass, and direct and indirect effects on bone metabolism. "Indeed, it is possible that the positive effect of estrogen on postmenopausal bone metabolism is in part mediated by activation of GH secretion."

But cautions Thorner, "That does not mean it's cause and effect."

Thorner told us in 1991, "I would argue that young women have much higher levels of GH than postmenopausal women and if you think that young women are healthier than old women, then it does not take a great leap of faith to say we should try and mimic what's happening in younger women."

But raising GH levels through estrogen has a number of side issues. Estrogen replacement in women is often used to relieve distressing symptoms of menopause, when they occur, and to guard against osteoporosis. Low doses of estrogen are safe and quite effective. The protection estrogen offers against bone loss is due in part to its synergy with GH. However, to get enough estrogen in the body to reestablish youthful levels of GH would require a lot more exogenous estrogen than is usually given to menopausal women. The reason for this, Thorner explains, is that with aging there may be a certain hypothalamic defect, that is, a deficiency of growth hormone releasing hormone (GHRH)—just as there very often is in GH-deficient children. Thus estrogen alone may not restore youthful GH levels.

High doses of estrogen are not good for women (let alone men) because of possible side effects. For one thing, estrogen, taken orally, unlike naturally secreted estrogen from the ovaries, goes relatively undiluted to the liver where it is degraded. The liver cells, you may recall, have many receptors for GH and, in response to GH, secrete Sm-C/IGF-I, the growth factor responsible for some of the indirect benefits of GH. The processing of estrogen in the liver is not without stress; it causes a degree of disruption of certain liver functions including its production of Sm-C/IGF. In fact, a substantial rise in GH has been observed with oral estrogen replacement but this positive effect has been accompanied by a lowering of Sm-C/IGF-I secretion.

The low Sm-C/IGF-I along with high GH may be explained by the system of feedback to the pituitary and the hypothalamus. The low Sm-C/IGF-I level in the blood carries a message back that the pituitary had better get cracking with more GH. The pituitary and hypothalamus have no way of knowing that the lowered Sm-C/IGF-I is not a result of low GH but of changes in the function of the liver as the result of estrogen.

But that's not all bad. Remember that GH produces its biological effects in tissues by a direct action, as well as indirectly via Sm-C/IGF-I. The enhanced GH secretion accompanying estrogen replacement may still produce *beneficial* effects directly in multiple peripheral tissue such as muscle and bone.

From the level of research in this area, it is clear there is much more to come in the saga of women, estrogen, and growth hormone.

GH and Fertility

A connection, however mysterious, between GH and estrogen brings up another subject of special interest to women: fertility. GH has been found in animal studies to increase the level of the growth factor Sm-C/IGF-I at the ovaries and to affect ovarian function. A pilot study reported in 1988 on eight women who had not been able to conceive and were being induced to ovulate by treatment with gonadotropins, that is, the pituitary hormones that stimulate the sex gland activity. Some of them were resistant to the treatment. When they were given GH along with the gonadotropins, however, ovarian response was increased and less gonadotropin over a shorter period of time was needed to induce ovulation. Thus GH treatment may provide a new method of inducing ovulation for in vitro fertilization or test tube babies as well as conception the regular way.

In 1988 Blumenfeld and Lunenfeld reported using GH to help a woman with multi-hypopituitarism who had been treated with gonadotropins for four cycles without conceiving. With GH she was treated with half the dose and got pregnant on the second cycle. The next year Volpe et al. used GH with gonadotropin-releasing hormone on an infertile 35-year-old woman. In due time she had twin boys. In sum, GH may make other fertility-enhancing hormone treatment doubly effective.

A few researchers in several countries have reported successful studies of using GH to facilitate ovulation in small numbers of women. However, long term studies of GH treatment on larger numbers of women are needed to determine optimum dosages, safety and efficacy. Much has been said, especially since the discovery in 1971 of serious problems associated with the synthetic hormone DES, about the long-term dangers of hormone treatment for infertility which often involves high doses and long periods of time. The use of GH for this purpose must undergo intense scrutiny for this very reason; on the other hand, by cutting down the need for high doses of other hormones and by getting the job done more quickly, GH may make the process of fertility therapy safer.

GH and Healing

Because of its restorative properties, growth hormone is being tried in a variety of situations where more rapid cell growth seems desired. In Norway in 1987, an elderly diabetic patient who already had one leg amputated and was getting around well on a prosthesis was hospitalized with a large, deep ulcer on the heel of his remaining foot. An orthopedist had recommended amputation of the foot, but the endocrinologist, Harald Waago, wanted to try one more thing to save the man's ability to walk. Waago made up an ointment of Vaseline (R) and codliver oil to which he added growth hormone. He applied this ointment off and on over the next month to the ulcer that had been growing wider and deeper over seven months of traditional treatment. During intermittent GH treatment, tissue destruction halted. In the next month with constant GH treatment, the ulcer diminished from an area of 40 square centimeters to an little blemish of less than one square centimeter. The foot was saved!

A fantastic feat that should bring hope to thousands of diabetics facing amputation? Well, maybe. But there was a fly in the ointment. The morning the patient was to be discharged, he was found dead in bed from a heart attack. And with just one patient in this "study," who could say for sure that the healing of the ulcer was more relevant than the heart attack? Also, during the treatment period, the patient's metabolism had stabilized. Maybe that, rather than GH, was the cure of the ulcer. A larger number of patients treated with GH would be needed to determine if GH has a role in treating this dreaded scourge of advanced diabetes, the relentless ulcer.

Later that year, Waago tried the same GH concoction on other patients. One diabetic woman, whose toe had to be amputated, had healed well for several days when the wound opened and grew worse. Leg amputation was considered but Waago was again given a chance to try GH. After a total of 58 days of treatment the wound was completely healed. Another elderly woman with an open pressure ulcer had four times rejected her surgeon's recommendation of amputation of her foot. The application of Waago's remedy for 65 days healed the ulcer and saved the foot. Word got around and several departments of the Tronheim hospital, including orthopedics and dermatology, began using GH. So did other Norwegian and Danish hospitals. But still there were no trials using larger numbers of patients. Finally, in 1991 Lars Rasmussen, of the Norwegian pharmaceutical company Novo Nordisk, and colleagues, authors of a study on 18 experimental subjects with chronic ulcers, reported a healing rate of 16% per week with GH treatment compared to 3% per week for the 11 controls. There were no side effects and no significant absorption of GH into the system. The latter point is especially important for diabetics because GH in the bloodstream tends to increase insulin intolerance, thereby worsening diabetes.

Waago has been disappointed that the Rasmussen group, like some of the clinical staff, would not use the cod liver oil, which Waago believes reduces the amount of GH necessary and reduces the huge cost of treatment. In 1990, however, he started a project to test his ointment, and at last Nordisk, a Norwegian pharmaceutical company which manufactures GH, has taken over sponsorship. Waago in 1992 started another double-blind project with American manufacturer, Eli Lilly, to treat pressure ulcers with Lilly's GH product, Humatrope.

In another experiment at Harvard Medical School, researchers studied the healing rates of patients who had patches of skin taken from one place on their bodies (donor sites) and grafted onto the site of a burn injury or ulcer. Eight skin graft patients were given daily injections of GH. Their skin graft donor sites healed approximately two days faster than the donor sites of the controls. Big deal? No, but this is how big deals start out. You have a small trial, little effect; a different dose, another trial, a hint of success; another trial following up on the hint; several more small trials, modifications; analysis of results of studies at other research centers, a larger trial...and so on...until break-through.

Besides the treatment of ulcers, GH is being tried experimentally, with different degrees of success, in a variety of situations in which more rapid cell growth is desirable, from healing burns to bone grafting.

GH and Physical Stress

The body's reaction to physical stress—an operation, injury, or infection, for example—is not just a local healing process but a systemic metabolic response, say James Manson and Douglas Wilmore in their summary article, "Growth Hormone and the Surgical Patient." These researchers explain, "One feature of the metabolic adaptation following stress is the mobilization of amino acids from skeletal muscle, the major site of body protein. The protein losses are minimal and well tolerated if the patient is healthy, body composition is normal, and the clinical course is normal. Following major burn injury, multiple trauma, or prolonged sepsis (infection), however, continued erosion of body protein and progressive loss of body nitrogen occur and result in protein malnutrition. In this situation the patient is unable to heal wounds and/or resist infection." (Loss or gain in protein reserves is regularly measured by the balance between nitrogen retention and nitrogen excretion.)

At first glance, the solution seems to be to feed the patient. Spoon it in or pipe it in, just get the protein in the body. Unfortunately, studies show that "feeding critically ill patients does not alter the accelerated rate of protein breakdown" and actually causes more stress. Very sick people can't digest food well and feeding tubes present their own problems. A better answer could be to modify the metabolic response to stress so that protein is better retained. And what agent is particularly known to stimulate protein synthesis? GH, of course.

In fact the role of GH in making the body use the fat stores and spare the muscle protein in times of stress has been an important one. The stresses of battle, hunt, famine, or other adversity increase GH secretion. (The figure on the next page illustrates the GH response to lack of food.) Over the centuries, the ability to maintain the muscle and use the fat stores has saved many a hungry, wounded hunter or warrior as he limped home. In modern times, investigators L. C. Carey and colleagues have studied soldiers seriously wounded in Vietnam. As soon as the injured arrived at the nearest medical base, the GH in their blood was measured at an average of five or six times normal, evidently a natural response to conserve strength in the form of protein reserves.

A similar surge of GH has also been noted following surgery, the more serious the operation the higher the GH. The ability to mount a GH response following injury, surgery, or other trauma apparently facilitates recovery. Unfortunately, however, the effect does not last more than a few days.

So extending and boosting the body's GH surge in

response to stress became the next order of business.

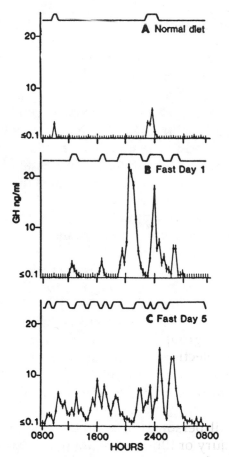

Serum GH levels measured every 20 minutes for 24 hours in a normal 37-year-old male prior to (A), during day 1 (B), and during day 5 (C) of a 5-day fast. Computer identification of GH pulses are shown above each profile. The shaded bars indicate integrated GH (μg minute/ml) of each of the 3 days. *From Thorner M.O., Vance M.L., Evans W.S., Blizzard R.M., Rogol A.D., Ho K., Leong D.A., Borges J.L.C., Cronin M.J., MacLeod R.M., Kovaks K., Asa S., Horvath E., Frohman L., Furlanetto R., Klingensmith G.J., Brook C., Smith P., Reichlin S., Rivier J. and Vale W.: "Physiological and Clinical Studies of GRF and GH."* Recent Progress in Hormone Research. *Used with permission of Academic Press.*

Ziegler et al. in 1988 gave GH injections to normal volunteers who, in order to simulate the nutritional deprivation of many patients, were allowed to consume only 60% of their calorie requirements. The nitrogen retention (hence protein retention) of the experimental patients increased with GH in spite of the cutback in food.

Recently a series of studies were conducted using patients hospitalized for major gastrointestinal surgery. Such patients by virtue of their original disorder are almost always physically "run-down"; after the trauma of surgery they have crucial need for nutrition to maintain body mass and for energy. In one study researchers Sim, Ward, Ponting, Teale, and Halliday at the Academic Surgical Unit at St. Mary's Hospital in London gave GH to a group of such patients before surgery; in the other studies the team gave the GH injections for the week following surgery. All studies showed improved utilization of nutrients measured primarily by a positive nitrogen balance. Moreover, Dahn et al., a group of several investigators who have given GH injections experimentally to post-surgical patients, have found that those who responded to GH treatment also had indications of increased immune response.

For a frail person who has been wasting away because of injury or illness, the GH treatment may lessen the trauma of surgery. Since the elderly make up a large percent of those undergoing serious surgery and since the elderly often are GH-deficient, it makes sense that these in particular may benefit from pre- or post-surgical GH administration.

GH and Dieting

Obesity is a threat to health and well-being for many

reasons. Moreover, obesity has been found to reduce GH secretion, so that just when a person most needs some of the hormone's benefits there is little to be found.

Treatment with exogenous GH seems a logical way to help obese people trying to lose weight because it turns the fuel into muscle instead of fat. Nobody, however, thinks you can inject growth hormone and then sit back and watch the fat melt away. Let's face it, losing weight, for the obese or even the slighty pudgy, depends primarily on eating less food. But the problem with eating less is that the resulting weight loss is accompanied in the obese by "an obligatory loss of muscle mass," according to David Clemmons and Louis Underwood, researchers at the University of North Carolina who have studied the process of losing fat while keeping the muscle. Serious weight loss is often accompanied by weakness and fatigue as well as measurable loss of protein.

Clemmons and Underwood have noted that the growth factor Sm-C/IGF-1, under the influence of both GH and nutrition, stimulates protein synthesis in muscle. When calories are restricted, Sm-C/IGF-I levels fall and muscle suffers. Here's where GH may help. Injections of GH do not make the fat drop off faster in most patients but short term GH therapy does help raise Sm-C/IGF-I levels and enhance protein retention during dieting. In other words, GH may help dieters stay on their feet.

Between Research and Practice...

When researchers study GH, Sm-C/IGF-I, nitrogen retention, and strength in the obese or postoperative cases, they are not yet at the point of helping fat people or saving surgical patients. Rather they are just trying to learn more about the mechanisms of metabolism. They will succeed at that, step by step. It is too early to say if their research will actually result in widespread GH therapy for the obese or for those facing surgery, for the weak and the elderly.

In the necessary gap between research and practice, people talk. The summer Rudman's study of GH therapy for elderly men made headlines, two aging baby-boomer couples were discussing the "less fat, more lean" results. George suggested: "Maybe we were never meant to mimic what's happening in younger people. Maybe older people were designed to have more fat for a good reason—like to keep them warm in their less active years."

"What!?!" exclaimed his wife, Bonnie, also pushing fifty. The other couple murmured their objections, too. They had no intention of acquiescing to passing years, they said. They plan to be playing tennis in their retirement years, not sitting in a rocking chair, and they'll do without the protective fat, thank you.

"That's what legwarmers are for," said Bonnie.

The others laughed. Still we know that the unwillingness of adults to sit back and let flesh crumble, sag, and go to paunch while GH is available is serious business.

In fact, some who beat a path to the door of the Baxamed Clinic in Basil, Switzerland, are being treated with GH as we speak. According to Marilyn Chase of the *Wall Street Journal*, founding physician Dr. Sam Baxas is also treating himself and his wife with human growth hormone to experience first hand its "youth-promoting" effects. Europe is more liberal in these matters than the U.S.

If GH-replacement is ever approved in the United States for the millions who may be deficient or even for a more general population, and especially if the GH or GH-stimulator of the future is more moderately priced and less unpleasant to take, beefing up with GH may become as common as washing away the gray.

CHAPTER THIRTEEN

GH and the Jock

A sharp grunt and then a long soulful sigh. More grunts and gasps follow in rhythmic pattern, building to evermore satisfying cries, and a final orgasmic release. The shaking stops; sweat trickles silently.

The workout is over. The body builder replaces his weights on their racks and towels off in the bright light streaming through high gymnasium windows. Bulges on arms and thighs glisten. Dark shadows define muscle mountains and ravines not softened by—dare we say the word?—fat. The ultimate triumph of lean.

Lean over fat. Where have we heard that before? Is that not the battle cry of growth hormone, its reason for being?

In September 1989 a national class body builder and owner of a gym in Carmichael, California, along with a companion, sold $100,000 worth of growth hormone, reportedly manufactured by Eli Lilly Co., to undercover agents. The drug is legally distributed only by a physician's prescription. The confiscated GH would have been worth something like $500,000 on the black market. This incident represented the first federal charges involving the illegal distribution of biosynthetic GH, a drug increasingly sought by top athletes and body builders as a substitute for anabolic steroids.

Anecdotal information circulating among the gym set says GH is as potent for building up and repairing muscle tissue under workout stress as steroids and has the added advantage that its use cannot be detected as yet in urine tests. (However, at least one company is working on the development of a urine test for GH detection.) GH is used certainly by only the top contenders as its costs—$600 to $1,200 per dose on the black market—are prohibitive. Rumor and reality have involved a few big names. Olympic Gold medalist Florence Griffith Joyner was accused, a year after the Olympics, of having taken GH. Another sprinter said he sold her 10 cubic centimeters of the drug for $2,000. Joyner denied buying or using the muscle builder. In the summer of 1991, a repentant Lyle Alzado, retired National Football League star, admitted to having added GH use to his long term steroid habit.

The Source

Bona fide GH is not readily manufactured in basement and back rooms labs because the process is difficult to set up and expensive to master. However, GH is acquired illicitly in several ways, according to Virginia Cowart, who follows athletic drug use issues. In a few cases, GH has been stolen directly from the drug companies in spite of security considerably tighter than that required by the FDA. In one notable case, a physician bought up a large quantity of GH and set up a marketing chain to resell it illegally. More often physicians "help" an athlete/client by prescribing the drug and accounting for it through false records. Some of the drug is imported from manufacturers in Europe. According to one account, foreign-made GH has been smuggled into the U.S. in ice cream containers so it would receive the refrigeration necessary to maintain potency. Where there is demand, there is supply. And where there is demand, there are also fakes. Some of the GH available on the black market is not the real thing but an unknown white crystalline substance with a counterfeit label.

Little Evidence of Abuse

In 1989, the United States General Accounting Office issued a report on the misuse of anabolic steroids and human growth hormone. The report found a big difference in the extent of abuse of steroids and growth hormone, citing only anecdotal evidence for growth hormone misuse. In addition, it noted less than 250 vials of purported human growth hormone were seized over a three-year period—this out of more than 1,500,00 vials shipped by the two FDA-approved marketers of recombinant growth hormone (Genentech and Eli Lilly) over approximately the same period. Of the purported human growth hormone seized, 42 percent was counterfeit.

While the GAO recommended greater federal and state controls for steroids, it made no such recommendation for human growth hormone. A federal law makes it a felony to distribute growth hormone for nonmedical uses. Many states have similar laws.

But Does GH Really Work for Muscle Builders?

Legality is only one of the issues surrounding the use of GH by athletes. Efficacy is also a major issue.

Did the clientele of the California body builder cum drug dealer get the results they paid for? Or did they just think they did? GH has been proven beyond a doubt to build muscle at the expense of fat for GH-deficient children; GH has also been proven in separate studies by Saloman and Rudman to alter the composition in favor of muscle for elderly GH-deficient men and by Crist et al. for sedentary GH-deficient women. But will it build muscle for those who already have enough GH and, even more relevant, for those who have reached a plateau of muscle development through athletic training?

Crist again has attempted to answer the question. He and his colleagues at the University of New Mexico studied the effects of the administration of biosynthetic GH on the body composition of well-trained, exercising young adults, men and women who had engaged in progressive resistance training, for example, weight lifting, for an average of over six years. The premise was that novices might get a quick fix of lean body mass—that is, muscle— from GH treatment but these jocks, who seemed maxed out on muscle already, might be another story. In the placebo-controlled, double-blind study, all subjects kept on eating the same high protein diet and pumping iron. They all experienced the GH treatment for six weeks and the placebo treatment for six weeks in random order. When the results were in, it was clear these folks all got even less fat and even more muscle with GH. How much of a change in body composition they experienced depended on dose. As might be expected, the GH-dependent growth factor Sm-C/IGF-I rose also during GH-treatment.

Thus it is reasonable to conclude that body builders or those who want more muscle bulk could get an edge over the competition from the anabolic effects of biosynthetic GH. With more GH, more muscle mass can be piled on.

Whether athletes, as opposed to body builders, can

enhance performance in speed, strength, or endurance, by taking supraphysiological (that is, higher than normal) doses of GH, however, is an entirely different question.

Muscle vs Performance

Muscles, those mounds and troughs of flesh that body builders show off, are generally an indication of strength. However, muscle mass put on by means of exogenous GH may not be the contractile kind, that is, the kind that can, by contracting, do work. To find out, strength must be measured distinct from muscle mass.

Of the few studies which have attempted to measure strength as a function of GH, we have already mentioned two. One by Hintz showed in preliminary results that grip strength was less in elderly people with lower Sm-C/IGF-I than in their agemates with more Sm-C/IGF-I, and the other by Cuneo showed that quadricep strength of GH-deficient adults was lower than that of normal controls. The link between lower strength and lower GH or Sm-C/IGF-I probably means that GH therapy would increase strength, but that is not proven. The observation of Robert Bensing, one of Rudman's elderly subjects, that he could open jars better after his treatment with GH is anecdotal, that is, it's the story Bensing told, but it was not scientifically documented. Remember, also, that Bensing was a GH-deficient subject given a dose of GH to bring him up to normal. Bensing's experience, if valid, would not necessarily indicate that a person with a normal level of GH secretion would become stronger with a supraphysiological level of GH.

Work- and hormone-induced muscle growth seem to be the result of two independent biochemical processes, says Bert Jacobson of Oklahoma State in a 1990 review, and, in fact, some investigators think that new tissue resulting from above-normal levels of GH does not contribute to strength. They base that conclusion on observations that acromegalics have muscle enlarged by increased muscle collagen, a non-contractile protein, accompanied by weakened muscle strength.

In spite of the uncertainty of experts about the strength-enhancing qualities of GH, athletes are risk-takers; they will try it if it might help performance. Athletic unions give credence to the belief that GH helps performance by banning the substance. The use of GH is banned by the U.S. Olympic Committee (USOC), the International Olympic Committee (IOC), and the National College Athletic Association (NCAA) in recognition of the idea that GH gives users unfair advantage.

The Down Side

Another finding of the Crist study is also of interest to those who might consider using GH illicitly for its anabolic effect. Five out of seven subjects secreted less endogenous GH than normal after the treatment with *exogenous* GH. That figures. The feedback loop that tells the hypothalamus that the GH level is sufficient probably detected the extra GH and signaled the pituitary to lay off production. The body in that way tends to resist supraphysiological levels. So for these individuals, if they were to routinely use GH as an anabolic drug, the first increment in GH would go to replenish the natural GH lost.

Moreover, growth hormone is dangerous when it is present in a level above normal for an extended period of time. Remember those acromegalic giants in Chapter Five? Not only were they big but they were deformed and unhealthy. Endocrinologists who have looked at photos of athletes around the world have sometimes recognized the acromegalic look, that is, the large features of the individual who has had too much growth hormone in his system for too long. While doctors who know the syndrome well can guess which athletes are long time GH abusers, they cannot positively identify them from one picture, because there is always the chance the guy with the bulging brow and nose and the jutting chin was destined by genes to look that way. However, several pictures over a period of years can confirm tissue changes that mark acromegaly and long term GH use. When a bony prominence of the face has enlarged or the fingers have widened noticeably, you can be sure that similar distortions are taking place inside the GH user's body.

Another problem with the illicit use of GH is that it may not be supervised by an ethical physician. That means especially that dosages may not be chosen with the well-being of the patient in mind. Donald Leggett of the FDA consumer safety office cites reports of athletes using twenty times the dose recommended for GH deficient children; all the power that is needed for making young kids grow, multiplied by twenty, would likely damage the heart of a normal person.

A third and by no means small problem of the illicit GH user is that the so-called GH available on the black market may be something else, and the supposedly sterile water packed with it may be tap water or contaminated water. A spokesman from Genentech says that the company, like Lilly also, tracks all of its sales and, when a drug bust is reported, samples and packaging are sent back to the manufacturer for identification and distribution records. Of all the reported seizures only a fraction actually involve bona fide products. You have only to look at the "quality control" of street drugs to guess what the quality of bootleg GH is. Even when the illicit GH is real, it may not have been kept cold as is necessary to preserve potency; if it's room temperature it's definitely bad. If it's cold to the touch there is still no guarantee it has been cold the whole trip from the manufacturer to the black market.

So, left to our own devices within the realm of safety and legitimacy, is there any way we adults can assure ourselves even adequate GH? Is there any way we could be, say, on the high end of normal? Could we get our body to manufacture more GH?

We remember that "Be Your Best (TM)" drink we were offered on the mall of the capital in Washington, and the body building amino acid supplements sold in the health food store. Ingredients like arginine and ornithine can boost your GH, the labels said. We remember these substances can, when injected, produce a surge of GH in a normal person and are used in stimulation tests for GH-deficiency for that very reason. So GH boosters in a pill are maybe something we should look into.

GH and Protein Supplements

We stopped by Natural Wonders of the World, the health food store in the nearest strip shopping center. While we browsed among shriveled umeboshi plums, dried lotus root, and Loveburger mix, we heard a slim young woman with a tennis headband and muscular tanned legs, saying, "I need to lose some of this fat. Have you got something to burn off the fat?"

"I've got arginine, ornithine, and lysine tablets," the clerk suggested.

"What's that?"

"They are amino acids that stimulate the brain to

produce more growth hormone," said the clerk. "That will give you more muscle and less fat."

"Will it work on my fanny?" the young woman asked.

The clerk gave an optimistic shrug.

On such a slight recommendation, she selected a jar of capsules from the Muscle Blaster Series and joined the leagues of athletes and would-be athletes who seek enhancement of their physique through protein supplement.

Of all the amino acids, the building blocks of proteins, only nine are not synthesized in the body and must come from our diet. Complete proteins, for example, albumin from eggs and casein from milk, contain all nine proteins in the right proportions. Individual vegetable proteins are incomplete but several together may comprise a complete protein also. Only the most stringent vegetarian diets would necessitate protein supplements for good health.

The recommended daily allowance (RDA) of protein for ordinary people is .8 grams per kilogram of body weight. Endurance athletes may need 50% to 100% more. Strength athletes also may need extra protein for muscling up. But the most any athlete should need per day, says Peter Lemon and colleagues at Kent State University, is 1.6 gm. per kilogram, or twice the RDA, that is, 100 grams for a 220-pound linebacker. A 1983 study of Syracuse University football players, however, revealed that the average protein intake from food was 200 grams a day or twice the maximum need. Certainly these athletes would not need additional protein, yet 18% of them took protein supplements anyway. The Syracuse players are apparently typical.

These athletes are hoping the excess proteins will pile up on their biceps, quadriceps, lats and pecs, although few scientific studies justify their hopes. Some athletes, body builders, and figure-conscious people like the lady at the health food store seek out certain protein supplements such as arginine, ornithine, and lysine because they know that in large quantities these amino acids specifically can give a boost to GH production. Each of these amino acids, in fact, has been administered by injection to stimulate a measurable GH surge for a test of GH sufficiency. Although the process of digestion breaks down complex proteins into simpler proteins, oral administration of these amino acids has a similar though lesser effect on GH levels.

However, University of Minnesota nutrition expert Joanne Slavin says of arginine supplements, "Most available supplements provide only milligram quantities of arginine and will not affect growth hormone release, which is fortunate in view of the potential dangers caused by an excess of GH." While we agree with Slavin's comment about the dangers of excessive GH, we must question her conclusion about the effect of available supplements on GH release. Let's look at the amounts of amino acids studies show are necessary to stimulate a GH surge; then let's compare those with amounts indicated on labels of supplements available in health food stores.

Isidori and colleagues in 1981 studied the rise of GH after oral administration of 1200 mg. of selected amino acid supplements. Blood tests at different times for two hours after administration showed the ingested amino acids caused a rise in GH similar to that stimulated by the same amino acids administered by injection: The 1200 mg. dose of arginine increased GH 185%, and the 1200 mg. of lysine increased GH 329%, a boost Bert Jacobson, Ed.D. of Oklahoma State University, calls "minimal." A combination of 1200 mg. of arginine and

1200 mg. of lysine together, however, caused a synergistic 794% increase. Interestingly, 2400 mg. of arginine taken orally resulted in a 278% drop in GH blood levels.

For comparison, our drink on the Washington mall, according to the label, contained 6 grams (6000 mg.) per serving of L. arginine (five times what caused a boost in the Isidori study and more than twice the amount that caused the bust).

We found at Natural Wonders, that one tablet of an Amino 1000 product labeled "performance nutrition" contained only 65.4 mg. of arginine, but it was combined with similar quantities of other GH-boosting amino acids and the directions said, "Take four to sixteen a day." A single-amino acid product contained 500 mg. of "free form" arginine per tablet; its label recommended one tablet per day or "as directed." Another supplement label was more specific, adding, "as directed by your trainer." Our fellow shopper who had complained of a fat fanny eventually chose a supplement called Firm Up whose label suggested taking "one or more capsules" and listed the contents of a 4-capsule dose as 1200 mg. arginine and 1200 mg. lysine, the same amounts and substances as Isidori et al. found gave a substantial GH jolt, plus 1200 mg. of ornithine. Clearly, a determined consumer may get enough of the amino acids to experience a GH surge like those in Isidori's study for less than 50 cents. There is no data to show that a temporary surge of that magnitude on a daily basis would change body composition. Undoubtedly, however, some athletes take large quantities of these supplements for that purpose—at the risk of putting their amino acid balance out of whack.

In the United States "health foods" including nutrition supplements are not regulated by the FDA. The FDA's Canadian counterpart, the Health Protection Branch, however, was concerned enough about misuse and overuse of amino acids that in the late 1980s it reclassified amino acids as drugs, suspending their across-the-counter sales during the testing period.

GH and Exercise

While we are looking at substances that are proven GH-stimulators, let's not overlook another stimulus that has also been used to provoke a GH surge during screening tests: vigourous exercise. It's cheap, it's safe, and it works.

No doubt about it, says University of Connecticut neurobiologist M. Deschenes after surveying studies on GH and exercise. The studies show that resistance training elevates GH, if it's intense enough. For example, in a 1988 study by W. Kraemer et al., when subjects exercising at 70% to 80% of their 1-repetition maximum resistance, their GH levels rose. However, when the resistance was lowered enough so subjects could do 21 repetitions, GH levels were unaffected.

Aerobic exercise can also increase GH secretion, the greater the intensity, the greater the GH surge. For example, in a 1986 study by W. Van Helder et al. in which subjects exercised on a bicycle ergometer at 40% of their maximum oxygen uptake (VO_2 max), their GH rose 145%; in a study the same year by P. Farrell and colleagues, subjects who exercised on a bicycle ergometer at 70% of their VO_2 max experienced a 166% rise in GH.

With different exercise protocols, the GH elevations lasted different lengths of time. In some studies, elevated GH levels dropped off as soon as exercise stopped. In others, the GH elevation lasted into the recovery period; in the Van Helder study, the maximum GH level was measured at 8 minutes after exercise stopped. There is no indication, however, that intense exercise raises resting GH levels.

Some studies show the effects of intense exercise on GH levels are less pronounced in well-trained individuals than in those who do not do strenuous exercise regularly. In other words, the worse shape you are in, the more you have to gain. Some studies also show that the effects of exercise on GH secretion may be greater in women than men.

In any case, there is, as yet, no way to measure how much a moderately elevated, short term GH surge contributes to the anabolic effects of exercise. Consider that runners experience GH elevation during runs of sufficient intensity but typically do not muscle up the way weight trainers do.

Running Rodents

Human runners might learn something from dedicated hamster runners, says researcher K.T. Borer, who has studied hamsters, running activity, and GH. "High volumes of spontaneous running are as puzzling in hamsters as in humans," Borer notes dryly. During his research, he observed that "footpads of running hamsters often show blisters and sores, yet the animals do not reduce their running in spite of such injuries. Determined distance runners are similarly reported to ignore discomfort and injuries."

Hamsters who run at night (hamsters are nocturnal), unlike their sedentary peers, had increased circulating GH in the morning. This finding was hardly unexpected from what we know about exercise and GH. Equally predictable was the finding that the running rodents experienced "absolute and relative increases in lean body mass and relative decreases in body fat content." But there's more: after a month of voluntary running, the hamster harriers showed significant lengthening of bones—even though these rodents were in adulthood.

Although such evidence of GH action is not readily applicable to humans, Borer does note reports of significant human bone growth in limbs used in sports extending even into young adulthood. He suggests that we should examine further the relationship of endurance exercise on growth in adolescents. Noting that intense endurance activity over a long period of time delays puberty in young girls, he suggests the possibility that "such exercise would at least extend the period of growth if not accelerate its rate as well."

It is very important to note here, however, that exercise accompanied by insufficient calories or inadequate nutrition decreases growth (in hamsters or humans) no matter what the GH status is. Sm-C/IGF-I secretion, though dependent on GH, is particularly sensitive to inadequate diet, falling rapidly when calorie intake does not support activity. This is sensible from the point of view of survival. When food supply is low, Sm-C/IGF-I is low and GH is high. The low Sm-C/IGF-I does two things: First, it stops growth stimulation, leaving what calories there are to produce energy for survival activities. Second, as a part of the hypothalamic/pituitary/receptor feedback system, it signals the production of more GH, which in turn favors the retention of muscle over fat so that the human will have the strength to seek more food. When food is again plentiful, Sm-C/IGF-I will rise, growth in the young can resume, and GH will stop working overtime.

Speaking of the hamster studies, in which nutrition was also an experimental variable, Borer says, you might expect voluntary running to decrease when there was a food deficit, but the opposite was true. The less food they had, the more the hamsters ran. Borer speculates that running around may be an instinctive response because it could lead hungry hamsters to new sources of food. Sometimes human runners, too, get caught up in extreme running patterns coupled with insufficient nutrition that results in a condition called anorexia athletica.

All in all, exercise is good for us, and some of this benefit is likely achieved through the enhanced GH secretion that accompanies intense exercise. Chances are that some other of the many changes brought about by exercise—increased heart rate and circulation, for example—may produce a climate in which surges of extra GH are well tolerated and desirable from a health standpoint. But it is unproven that greater than normal levels of GH through injection or other chemical stimulation achieves an improvement in strength, fitness, or well-being of normal people. It is possible that long term higher-than-normal levels of GH will have just the opposite effect.

As ever, balance is the key to an optimum physical state: balance between energy expenditure and nutrition, between amino acids and other nutrients, and between too little GH and too much.

A Parting Toast

To Growth hormone...

- without which little children stay little and grown-ups grow frail...

- so powerful that a nanogram will set forces in motion all over the body, yet slave to the hypothalamus...

- precious in its effects, fabulous in its price...

- once bequeathed by the dead, now created by the humblest of bacteria in the cauldrons of industry...

- once rationed out, now unlimited, its uses expanding...

- still mysterious element in an intricate order of receptors, releasers, inhibitors...

- instigator of the moments of growth in which cells differentiate, multiply, synthesize...

- malignant in excess, boon to well-being in balance...

- a magic potion to be used with the care of a wizard.

REFERENCES

CHAPTER ONE

Haney D.: Hormone, a shot in the arm for fight on aging. *Chicago Sun-Times*, July 5, 1990.

Jorgensen J.O.L., Theusen L., Ingemann-Hansen T., Pedersen S.A., Jorgensen J., Skakkebaek N.E., Christiansen J.S.: Beneficial effects of growth hormone treatment in GH-deficient adults. *The Lancet*, 1989, June 3: pp. 1221-1225.

Lee M.: New Hope for elderly: Growth hormone restores strength. *Chicago Tribune*, July 5, 1990.

Peterson C.: 72-year-old tries 'elixir of life' in aging project. *The News-Sun*, (Waukegan, Illinois) July 11, 1990.

Random House Dictionary of the English Language. Stein, J., editor. Random House, New York: 1973.

Rudman D., Feller A., Nagraj H., Gergans G., Lalitha P., Goldberg A., Schlenker R., Cohn L., Rudman I., Mattson D.: Effects of human growth hormone in men over 60 years. *The New England Journal of Medicine*, 1990, vol. 323, July 5: pp. 1-6.

Salomon F., Cuneo R.C., Hesp R., Sonksen P.H.: The effects of treatment with recombinant human growth hormone on body composition and metabolism in adults with growth hormone deficiency. *The*

New England Journal of Medicine, 1989, vol. 321, no. 26; pp. 1797-1803.

Vance M.: Growth hormone for the elderly? *The New England Journal of Medicine*, 1990, vol. 323, July 5: pp. 52-54.

CHAPTER TWO

Goodgame D.: *Time Magazine*, May 1991.

Montgomery D.A.D. and Welbourne R.B.: *Medical and Surgical Endocrinology*. Edward Arnold Ltd., London, 1975.

Muthe N.C.: *Endocrinology: A Nursing Approach*. Little Brown and Co., Boston, 1981.

Plowman P.N.: *Endocrinology and Metabolic Diseases*. John Wiley and Sons Ltd., Sussex, U.K., 1987.

CHAPTER THREE

Medvei, V.C.: *A History of Endocrinology*. MTP Press, Lancaster & Boston 1982: 913 pages.

Brooks C., Gilbert J.L., Levey H.A., and Curtis D.R.: *Humors, Hormones, and Neurosecretions*. State University of New York, N.Y., 1962: 313 pages.

CHAPTER FOUR

Anderson S.H.: Obituaries, Choh Hao Li. *New York Times*, December 2, 1987.

Brazeau P., Vale W., Burgus R., Ling N., Butcher M., Rivier J., and Guillemin R.: Hypothalimic polypeptide that inhibits the secretion of immunoreactive pituitary growth hormone. *Science*, 1973, vol. 179: p.77.

Furlanetto R.W.: Insulin-like growth factor measurements in the evaluation of growth hormone secretion. *Hormone Research,* 1990, vol. 33, suppl. 4: pp. 25-30.

Hall R.: *The Lancet,* 1973, vol. 2: p. 581.

Ho K.K.: Evans W.S., Blizzard R.M., Veldhuis J.D., Merriam G.R., Samojlik E., Furlanetto R., Rogol A.D., Kaiser D.L., Thorner M.O.: Effects of sex and age on the 24-hour profile of growth hormone secretion in man: Importance of endogenous estradiol concentrations. *Journal of Clinical Endocrinology and Metabolism,* 1987; vol. 64, no.1; pp.51-58.

Laron Z. and Bauman B.: Growth hormone releasing hormone (GH-RH, GRF)—an important new clinical tool. *European Journal of Pediatrics,* 1986, vol. 145: p. 6-9.

Maugh T.H.: Obituaries, Choh Hao Li. *Los Angeles Times,* December 2, 1987.

Medvei, V.C.: *A History of Endocrinology.* MTP Press, Lancaster & Boston, 1982: 913 pages.

Muller E.E.: Clinical implications of growth hormone feedback mechanisms. *Hormone Research,* 1990; vol. 33, suppl. 4; pp. 90-96.

San Francisco Chronicle, Obituaries, Choh Hao Li. December 2, 1987.

Underwood L.E., editor: *Human Growth Hormone, Progress and Challenges.* Marcel Dekker, Inc., New York and Basel, 1988.

Vance M.L., Kaiser D.L., Martha P.M., Furlanetto R.W., Rivier J, Vale W., and Thorner M.O.: Lack of in vivo somatotroph desensitization or depletion after 14 days of continuous growth hormone (GH)-releasing hormone administration in normal men and a GH-deficient boy. *Journal of Clinical Endocrinology and Metabolism,* 1989, vol. 68, no. 1: pp. 22-28.

Vanderschueren-Lodeweyckx M.: Assessment of growth hormone secretion: What are we looking for practically? *Hormone Research*, 1990, volume 33, suppl. 4: pp. 1-6.

CHAPTER FIVE

Carlson, H.E.: Functioning Pituitary Tumors. *Practical Endocrinology*, Hershman J.M., editor. John Wiley and Sons and Medical Education Assoc., 1981.

Guinness Book of World Records. Russell A. and McWhirter N., editors. 1988, Sterling Publishing Co., N.Y.

Medvei, V.C.: *A History of Endocrinology*. MTP Press, Lancaster & Boston, 1982: 913 pages.

Melmed S., Ezrin K., Goodman R., and Frohman L.: Acromegaly due to secretion of growth hormone by an ectopic pancreatic islet-cell tumor. *New England Journal of Medicine*, 1985, vol. 312, no. 1: pp. 9-17.

Montgomery D.A.D. and Welbourn R.B.: *Medical and Surgical Endocrinology*. Williams and Wilkins Co., Baltimore.

New York Times: Marfan Syndrome news, May 3, 1991.

New York Times: Flo Hyman news, Feb. 5, 1988, sec. B.: p. 15.

Parks, J.S.: Evaluating tall stature. In Hurst, J.W., *Medicine for the Practicing Physician*, Butterworth Publishers, Boston, 1981.

Penney D.G., Dunbar J.C., and Baylerian M. S.: Cardiomegaly and haemodynamics in rats with a transplantable growth hormone-secreting tumor. *Cardiovascular Research*, 1985, vol. 19: pp. 270-277.

Rizza R.A., Mandarino L.J., and Gerich J.E.: Effects of

growth hormone on insulin action in man. *Diabetes*, 1982, vol. 31: pp. 663-669.

Wass J.A.H.: Octreotide treatment of acromegaly. *Hormone Research*, 1990; vol 33, suppl. 1: pp. 1-6.

CHAPTER SIX

Cross H.R.: *The Real Tom Thumb*. 1980, Four Wives Press, N.Y.

Grimm Brothers: *Grimm's Fairy Tales, Twenty Stories*. The Viking Press, New York, 1973.

Guinness Book of World Records. Russell A. and McWhirter N., editors. 1988, Sterling Publishing Co., N.Y.

Laron Z., Kelijman M., Pertzelan A., Keret R., Shoffner J.M., and Parks J.S.: Human growth hormone gene deletion without antibody formation or growth arrest during treatment—A new disease entity? *Israel Journal of Medical Sciences*, 1985, vol. 21: pp. 999-1006.

Zarin C.: A Part in the Play. *The New Yorker*, July 30, 1990: pp. 37-56.

CHAPTER SEVEN

August G.P., Lippe B.M., Blethen S.L., Rosenfeld R.G., Seelig S.A., Johanson A.J., Compton P.G., Frane J.W., McClellan B.H., and Sherman B.M.: Growth hormone treatment in the United States: Demographic and diagnostic features of 2331 children. *Journal of Pediatrics*, June, 1990: pp. 899-903.

Bierich J.R.: Multicentre Clinical trial of authentic recombinant somatropin in growth hormone deficiency. *Acta paediatrica Scandinavica*, 1987, vol. 337: pp. 135-140.

Colle M., Frangin G., Auzerie J., Ruffie A., Ruedas E.: A placebo-controlled trial of intranasal growth hormone-releasing hormone GHRH (1-44—NH) administration in normal young adults. *Hormone Research*, 1990, vol. 33: pp.1-4.

Costin G., Kaufman F.R., and Brasel J.A.: Growth hormone secretory dynamics in subjects with normal stature. *Journal of Pediatrics*, 1989, vol. 115, no. 4: pp. 537-544.

Darendeliler R., Hindmarsh P.C., and Brook C.G.D.: Dose-response curves for treatment with biosynthetic human growth hormone. *Journal of Endocrinology*, 1990, vol. 125: pp. 311-316.

Eli Lilly and Company. Humatrope (R) package insert. Indianapolis, Indiana.

Frasier S.D.: Human pituitary growth hormone (hGH) therapy in growth hormone deficiency. *Endocrine Reviews*, 1983, vol. 4, no. 2.

Frasier S.D.: A review of growth hormone stimulation tests in children. *Pediatrics*, 1974, vol. 53, no. 6.: pp. 929-936.

Genentech ,Inc. Protropin package insert. San Francisco, CA, 1985.

Hindmarsh P.C., Stanhope R., Preece M.A., Brook C.G.D.: Frequency of administration of growth hormone—an important factor in determining growth response to exogenous growth hormone. *Hormone Research*, 1990, vol. 33, suppl. 4: pp. 83-89.

Holcomb J.H., Wong A.C., Conforti J.J. et al.: Effect of an increased dose of somatropin in previously treated growth-hormone deficient children. *Pediatric Research*, 1989, vol. 25, no. 4, part 2, abstract no. 494.

Howrie D.: Growth hormone for the treatment of growth failure in children. *Clinical Pharmacy*, 1987, vol. 6, April: pp 283-291.

Job J-C: Results of long-term growth hormone replacement therapy in children: when and how to treat? *Hormone Research*, 1990, vol. 33, suppl. 4: pp. 69-76.

Jorgensen J.O.L., Moller J., Moller N., Lauritzen T., and Christiansen J.S.: Pharmacological aspects of growth hormone replacement therapy: route, frequency, and timing of administration. *Hormone Research*, 1990, vol. 33, suppl. 4: pp. 77-82.

Parks J.S.: Short stature and delayed puberty: Criteria for diagnosis. In Hurst, J.W., *Medicine for the Practicing Physician*, Butterworth Publishers, Boston, 1981.

Reiter E.O. and Martha P.M.: Pharmacological testing of growth hormone secretion. *Hormone Research*, 1990, vol. 33: pp. 121-127.

Rochiccioli P., Dechaux E., Tauber M.T., Pienkowski C., Tiberge M.: Growth hormone treatment in patients with neurosecretory dysfunction. *Hormone Research*, 1990, vol. 33, suppl. 4: pp. 97-101.

Rose S.R., Ross J.L., Uriarte M., Barnes K.M., Cassorlan F., and Cutler G.B.: The advantage of measuring stimulated as compared with spontaneous growth hormone levels in the diagnosis of growth hormone deficiency. *New England Journal of Medicine*, 1988; vol. 319, pp. 201-207.

Rosenbaum M., Gertner J., and Leibel R.: Effects of systemic growth hormone (GH) administration on regional adipose tissue distribution and metabolism in GH-deficient children. *Journal of Clinical Endocrinology and Metabolism*, 1989, vol. 69; no. 6.

Rosenblum A.L. and Knuth C.L.: Growth response of

growth hormone deficient patients to 0.06 mg/kg compared with 0.10 mg/kg three times per week of biosynthetic growth hormone. *AJDC*, 1989, vol. 143: pp. 642-643.

Spiliotis B.E., August C.P., Hung W., Sonis W., Mendelson W., and Bercu B.B.: Growth hormone neurosecretory dysfunction: A treatable cause of short stature. *Journal of American Medical Association*, 1984, vol. 251: pp. 2223-2230.

Stahnke N. and H. Koehn: Replacement therapy in hypo-thalamus-pituitary insufficiency: Management in the adolescent. *Hormone Research,* 1990, suppl. 4: pp. 38-44.

Tanner J.M.: Introduction, Growth hormone therapy, the target for a successful treatment. *Clinical Sequel No. 2,* 1986, Genentech, Inc.

Tanaka T., Yoshizawa A., Tanae A., Hibi I., Shizume K.: Relationships between puberty and growth at adolescence in growth-hormone-deficient males: Effect of growth hormone and of associated gonadal suppression therapy. *Hormone Research,* 1990, vol. 33, suppl. 4: 102-105.

Thorner M., et al.: Treatment of two children with GHRH: acceleration of growth. *New England Journal of Medicine,* 1985; vol. 312: pp. 4-9.

Van Vliet G., Bosson D., Robyn C., Craen M., Malvaux P., Vanderschuere-Lodeweyckx M., and Wolter R.: Effect of growth hormone releasing hormone on plasma growth hormone, prolactin, and somatomedin-C in hypopituitary and short normal children. *Hormone Research,* 1985, vol. 22: pp. 32-45.

Vanderschueren-Lodeweyckx M.: Assessment of growth hormone secretion: What are we looking for practically? *Hormone Research,* 1990, volume 33, suppl. 4: pp. 1-6.

CHAPTER EIGHT

Carney B.: Short Stuff! 1991; unpublished.

CHAPTER NINE

Allen B.A. and Fost N.C.: Growth hormone therapy for short stature: Panacea or Pandora's box? *Journal of Pediatrics,* 1990, vol. 117, no.1, part I: pp 16-21.

Bierich J.R.: Therapy with growth hormone—old and new indications. *Hormone Research,* 1989, vol 32: pp. 153-165.

Darendeliler F., Hindmarsh P.C., Brook C.G.D.: Nonconventional use of GH: European experience. *Hormone Research,* 1990, vol. 33: pp. 128-137.

Gertner J.M., Genel M., Gianfredi S.P., Hintz R.L., Rosenfeld R.G., Tamborlane W.V., and Wilson D.M.: Prospective clinical trial of human growth hormone in short children without growth hormone deficiency. *Journal of Pediatrics,* 1984, vol. 104, no. 2: pp. 172-176.

Godowski P.J., Leung D.W., Meacham L.R., Galgani J.P., Hellmiss R., Keret R., Rotwein P.S., Parks J.S., Laron Z., and Wood W.I.: Characterization of the human growth hormone receptor gene and demonstration of a partial gene deletion in two patients with Laron-type dwarfism. *Proceedings of the National Academy of Science USA,* 1989, vol. 86: pp. 8083-8087.

Kolata G.: New growth industry in human growth hormone? *Science,* 1986, vol. 234, October: pp. 22-24.

Linder B. and Cassoria F.: Short stature: Etiology, diagnosis, and treatment. *Journal of the American Medical Association*, 1988, vol. 260, no. 21: pp. 3171-3175.

Linder B., Feuillan P., and Chrousos G.P.: Alternate day prednisone therapy in congenital adrenal hyperplasia: Adrenal androgen suppression and normal growth. *Journal of Clinical Endocrinology and Metabolism*, 1989; vol. 69, no. 1: pp. 191-195.

Lippe B. and Frasier S.D.: How should we test for growth hormone deficiency, and whom should we treat? *Journal of Pediatrics*, 1989, vol. 115, no. 4: pp. 585-587.

Lantos J., Siegler M., Cuttler L.: Ethical issues in growth hormone therapy. *Journal of American Medical Association*, 1989, vol. 261, no. 7: pp. 1020-1024.

Mehis O. and Fine R.N.: The use of human recombinant growth hormone for treatment of growth failure in uremia. *Seminars in Nephrology*, 1989, vol. 9, no. 1: pp. 43-48.

Powell D.R.: Growth failure in children with chronic renal failure. *The Kidney*, 1989, vol. 22, no. 2: pp. 7-12.

Rosenfeld R.G.: Non-conventional growth hormone therapy in Turner Syndrome: The U.S. experience. *Hormone Research*, 1990, vol. 33: pp. 137-140.

Ross J.L., Long L.M., Loriaux D.L., Cutler G.B.: GH secretory dynamics in Turner Syndrome. *Journal of Pediatrics*, vol. 106, no. 2: pp. 202-206.

Tanaka T., Hibi I., and Shizume K.: GH secretion capacity in Turner syndrome and its influence on the effect of GH treatment. *Turner Syndrome: Growth Promoting Therapies.* M.B. Ranke and R.G. Rosenfeld, editors. Elsevier Science Publishers, B.V., 1991.

Tonshoff B., Mehls O., Schauer A., Heinrich U., Blum

W., and Ranke M.: Improvement of uremic growth failure by recombinant human growth hormone. *Kidney International*, 1989, vol. 36, suppl. 27: pp. S-201 - S-204.

Tonshoff B., Schauer A., Ranke M., Blum W., Heinrich U., and Mehls O.: Improvement of growth by recombinant human growth hormone in uraemic children. *Acta Paediatrica Scandinavia*, 1989, suppl. 349: p. 160.

Werth B.: How short is too short. *The New York Times Magazine*, June 16, 1991.

CHAPTER ELEVEN

Asbury C.: The orphan drug act, The first 7 years. *Journal of the American Medical Association*, 1991, vol. 265, no. 7: pp. 893-897.

Black W: Drug products of recombinant DNA technology. *American Journal of Hospital Pharmacy*, 1989, vol. 46, no. 9: pp. 1834-1844.

Cowart V.S.: Human growth hormone: The latest ergogenic aid? *The Physician and Sportsmedicine*, 1988; vol. 16, pp. 175-185.

Eli Lilly and Company. Humatrope (R) package insert. Indianapolis, Indiana.

Genentech, Inc. Protropin package insert. San Francisco, CA, 1985.

Okada Y., Taira K., Takano K., and Hizuka N.: A case report of growth attenuation during methionyl human growth hormone treatment. *Endocrinol. Japon*, 1987, vol. 34, no. 4: 621-626.

Root A.W.: Summing-up of symposium update on hGH: Clinical aspects. *Hormone Research*, 1990, vol. 33: p. 143.

Werth B.: How short is too short. *The New York Times Magazine*, June 16, 1991.

CHAPTER TWELVE

Aloia, John, Vaswani A., Meunier P., Edouard C., Arlot M., Yeh J., Cohn S.: Coherence treatment of postmenopausal osteoporosis with growth hormone and calcitonin. *Calcified Tissue International*, 1987, vol. 40: pp. 253-259.

Ammann, Arthur: Growth hormone and immunity. *Human Growth Hormone*. Louis Underwood, editor. Marcel Dekker,Inc., New York & Basel, 1988.

Bengtsson B., Brummer R., Bosaeus I.: Growth hormone and body composition. *Hormone Research*, 1990, vol. 33, suppl. 4: pp. 19-24.

Blumenfeld Z., Lunenfeld B.: The potentiating effect of growth hormone on follicle stimulation with human menopausal gonadotropin in a panhypopituitary patient. *Fertility and Sterility*, 1989, vol. 52, no. 2: pp. 328-331.

Chase, M.: Scientists work to slow human aging. *Wall Street Journal*. March 12, 1992, Sec. B, p.1.

Christiansen, J. Sandahl: Effects of growth hormone on body composition in adults. *Hormone Research*, 1990; vol. 33, suppl. 4: pp. 61-64.

Clemmons D.R., Synder K.K., Williams R., and Underwood L.E.: Growth hormone administration conserves lean body mass during dietary restriction in obese subjects. *Journal of Clinical Endocrinology and Metabolism*, 1987, vol. 64: pp. 878-883.

Crist D.M., Peake G.T., Mackinnon L.T., and Kraner J.C.: Exogenous growth hormone (GH) treatment alters body composition and increases natural killer cell activity in women with impaired endogenous GH secretion. *Metabolism Clinical Experiments*, 1987, vol. 36: pp. 1115-1117.

Cuneo R.C., Salomon F., Wiles C.M., Sonksen P.H.: Skeletal muscle performance in adults with growth hormone deficiency. *Hormone Research*, 1990, vol. 33, suppl. 4: pp. 55-60.

Dahn M.S., Mitchell R.A., Smith S.A. et al.: Altered immunological function and nitrogen metabolism associated with depression of plasma growth hormone. Journal of P.E.N., 1984, vol. 8: pp. 690-694.

Flynn, Margaret Nolph G.B., Baker A.S., Martin W.M., Krause G.: *American Journal of Clinical Nutrition*, 1989, vol. 50: pp. 713-717.

Hintz R.: Growth hormone, the somatomedins, and aging. *Human Growth Hormone*, Louis Underwood, editor; Marcel Dekker Inc., New York and Basel, 1988: pp. 219-229.

Ho K.Y., Evans W.S., Blizzard R.M., Veldhuis J.D., Merriam G.R., Samojlik E., Furlanetto R., Rogol A.D., Kaiser D.L., Thorner M.O. Effects of sex and age on the 24-hour profile of growth hormone secretion in man: Importance of endogenous estradiol concentrations. *Journal of Clinical Endocrinology and Metabolism*, 1987, vol. 64, no. 1: pp. 51-58.

Homburg R., Eshel A., Abdalla H.I., Jacobs H.S. Growth hormone facilitates ovulation induction by gonadotrophins. *Clinical Endocrinology*, 1988, vol. 29: pp. 113-117.

Jorgensen J.O.L., Theusen L., Ingemann-Hansen T., Pedersen S.A., Jorgensen J., Skakkebaek N.E., Christiansen J.S. Beneficial effects of growth hormone treatment in GH-deficient adults. *The Lancet*, 1989, June 3; pp. 1221-1225.

Marcus R., Butterfield G., Holloway L., Gilliland L., Baylink D.J., Hintz R.L., Sherman B.M.: Effects of short term administration of recombinant human growth hormone to elderly people. *Journal of Clinical Endocrinology and Metabolism*, 1990, vol. 70, no. 2: pp. 519-526.

McGauley G.A., Cuneo R.C., Saloman F., Sonksen P.H.: Psychological well-being before and after growth hormone treatment in adults with growth hormone deficiency. *Hormone Research*, 1990, vol. 33, suppl. 4: pp. 52-54.

Ponting G.A., Teale J.D., Halliday D., Sim A.J.W. Postoperative positive nitrogen balance with intravenous hyponutrition and growth hormone. *The Lancet*, 1988, February 27: pp 438-439.

Rasmussen L., Karlsmark T., Avnstorp C., Peters K., Jorgensen M., Jensen L. Topical human growth hormone treatment of chronic leg ulcers. *Phlebology*, 1991, vol. 6: pp. 23-30.

Rudman, Daniel, et al. Effects of human growth hormone in men over 60 years old. *New England Journal of Medicine*, 1990, vol. 323: p. 1.

Rudman, Daniel: Growth Hormone, Body Composition, and Aging. *Journal of the American Geriatrics Society*, Nov. 1985: pp. 800-807.

Rudman D., Kutner M.H., Rogers C.M., Lubin M.F.,Fleming G.A., Bain R.P. Impaired growth hormone secretion in the adult population. *American Society for Clinical Investigation*, 1981, vol. 67: pp. 1361-1369.

Salomon F., Cuneo R.C., Hesp R., Sonksen P.H. The effects of treatment with recombinant human growth hormone on body composition and metabolism in adults with growth hormone deficiency. *The New England Journal of Medicine*, 1989, vol. 321, no. 26: 1797-1803.

Shuster S., Black M., McVitie E. *British Journal of Dermatology*, 1975, vol. 93: pp. 639-643.

Sim A.J.W., Ward H.C., Ponting G.A., Teale J.D., Halliday D. Influence of hormones on post-operative metabolic responses with special reference to growth hormone. *The British Journal of Clinical Practice*, suppl 63: pp. 126-132.

Sonksen P.H.: Replacement therapy in hypothalamo-pituitary insufficiency after childhood: Management in adults. *Hormone Research*, 1990, vol. 33, suppl. 4: pp. 45-51.

Thorner M.O., Vance M.L., Evans W.S., Blizzard R.M., Rogol A.D., Ho K., Leong D.A., Borges J.L.C., Cronin M.J., MacLeod R.M., Kovaks K., Asa S., Horvath E., Frohman L., Furlanetto R., Klingensmith G.J., Brook C., Smith P., Reichlin S., Rivier J., and Vale W.: Physiological and clinical studies of GRF and GH. Recent Progress in Hormone Research, 1986; vol. 42, pp. 589.

Volpe A., Coukos G., Artini P.G., Silferi M., Petraglia F., Boghen M., D'Ambroglio G., Genazzani A.R. Pregnancy following combined growth hormone— pulsatile GnRH treatment in a patient with hypothalamic amenorrhea. *Human Reproduction*, 1990, vol. 5: pp. 345-347.

Waago, Harald. Local treatment of ulcers in diabetic foot with human growth hormone. (Letter) *The Lancet*, June 27, 1987: p. 1485.

Ward H.C., Halliday D., Sim A.J.W.: Protein and energy metabolism with biosynthetic human growth hormone after gastrointestinal surgery. *Annals of Surgery*, 1987, vol. 206, no. 1: pp. 56-61.

CHAPTER THIRTEEN

Borer K.T. Exercise-induced facilitation of pulsatile growth hormone secretion and somatic growth. *Hormones and Sport*, Laron Z. and Rogol A.D. Serono Symposia Publications from Raven Press, vol. 55: 1988.

Cowart V.S. Human growth hormone: The latest ergogenic aid? *The Physician and Sportsmedicine*, 1988, vol. 16: pp. 175-185.

Crist D., Peake G., Egan P., Waters D. Body composition response to exogenous GH during training in highly conditioned adults. The American Physiology Society, 1988: pp. 579-584.

Cuneo R.C., Salomon F., Wiles C.M., Sonksen P.H.: Skeletal muscle performance in adults with growth hormone deficiency. *Hormone Research* 1990, vol. 33, suppl. 4: pp. 55-60.

Deschenes M.R., Kraemer W.J., Maresh C.M., Crivello J.F. Exercise-induced hormonal changes and their effects upon skeletal muscle tissue. *Sports Medicine*, 1991, vol. 12, no. 2: pp. 85-93.

Hintz R. Growth hormone, the somatomedins, and aging. *Human Growth Hormone*. Louis Underwood, editor. Marcel Dekker, Inc., New York & Basel, 1988.

Isidori A., Lo Monaco A., and Cappa M. A study of growth hormone release in man after oral administration of amino acids. *Current Medical Research Opinion*, 1981, vol. 7, no. 7: pp. 475-481.

REFERENCES

Jacobson B.H. Effects of amino acids on growth hormone release: Growth Hormone. *The Physician and Sportsmedicine*, 1990, vol. 18, no. 1: pp. 63-70.

Kelly P.J., Eisman J.A., Stuart M.C., Pocock N.A., Sambrook P.N., and Gwinn T.H. Somatomedin-C, Physical Fitness, and Bone Density. *Journal of Clinical Endocrinology and Metabolism*, 1990, vol. 70, no. 3: pp. 718-723.

Los Angeles Times, September 28, 1989, Sec. 1: p. 3.

Merimee T.J., Rabinowitz M.D., and Fineberg S.E. Arginine-initiated release of human growth hormone: factors modifying the response in normal man. *New England Journal of Medicine*, 1969, vol. 280, no. 26: pp. 1484-1438.

Lemon P.W. and Proctor D.N.: Protein Intake and Athletic performance. *Sports Medicine*, 1991, vol. 12, no. 5: pp. 313-325.

Macintyre J.: Growth hormone and athletes. *Sports Medicine*, 1987, vol. 4, no. 2: pp. 129-142.

Rudman D., Feller A., Nagraj H., Gergans G., Lalitha P., Goldberg A., Schlenker R., Cohn L., Rudman I., Mattson D. Effects of human growth hormone in men over 60 years. *The New England Journal of Medicine*, 1990, vol. 323, July 5: pp. 1-6.

Salomon F., Cuneo R.C., Hesp R., Sonksen P.H. The effects of treatment with recombinant human growth hormone on body composition and metabolism in adults with growth hormone deficiency. *The New England Journal of Medicine*, 1989, vol. 321, no. 26: 1797-1803.

Slavin J., Lanners G., Engstrom M.: Amino Acid Supplements: Beneficial or Risky? *The Physician and Sportsmedicine*, 1988, vol. 16, no. 3: pp. 221-224.

United States General Accounting Office: "Drug Misuse: Anabolic Steroids and Human Growth Hormone." August 18, 1989.

Wagner J.: Enhancement of athletic performance with drugs: An overview. *Sportsmedicine*, vol. 12, no. 4: pp. 250-265.

INDEX

Abel, John Jacob, 50
achondroplasia, 113, 190-191
acromegaly, 73, 89-103, 123, 168, 187, 256; athletes and, 256-257; diagnosis of, 101-102; enlargement of organs in, 95; and folk literature, 97-98, 99; in history, 98-100; life span of people with, 95; mild, 100; role of pituitary in, 99-100; and scoliosis, 96; symptoms of, 89-91, 92-94, 96; treatment of, 102-103
Addison's disease, 47
Addison, Thomas, 47
adenoma *see* pituitary tumor
adrenal cortex, 32-33, 69, 95; hormones, 32-33, 69
adrenal glands, 21, 23, 31, 47, 49, 228; diseases of, 47, 87; extract and blood pressure, 50; hyperactive, 87-88; tumors, 87, 188

adrenalin, 23-26, 31-32, 38, 50, 51; effects of, 24, 25-26, 31-32; rush of, 24, 25-26, 31-32
adrenal medulla, 25, 31, 57; hormones, 31-32, 38
adrenocorticotrophic hormone (ACTH), 59, 65, 125-126
adults, 19; GH-deficient, 16, 226-229, 230-233; symptoms of GH-deficient, 226-229
androgen, 32, 38
aging, effects of, on body, 229-232; and GH-deficiency, 232-233
aldosterone, 32
Allen, David B., 166, 194-195, 196
Allen, Sandy, 78-79
Alzado, Lyle, 252
amino acids, 18-19, 218, 219, 258-259, 260-262
anabolic steroids, 177, 252, 253, 256
Anavar, 177

Anderson, Stephen, 125-126, 139, 193, 207-208
anorexia athletica, 193, 265
arginine, 18, 19, 124, 258, 260-261
Aristotle, 40
arthritis, 96
Aschner, Bernhard, 56-57
asthma, 188
athletes, 17; and acromegaly, 256-257; and GH use, 251-265

Barnum, Phineas T., 109, 110
Barry, Martin, 51
Baxas, Sam, 249
Baxter, Scott, 165-166
Beckwith-Wiedemann Syndrome, 87
Bengtsson, Bengt-Ake, 226
Bensing, Robert, 11-15, 255
Berthold, Arnold, 44-46
Bierich, J.R., 133, 179, 183, 184, 188
blood pressure, 25-26, 50; and adrenal extract, 50
bone age, 118, 127, 179, 181, 182, 185, 188, 189, 202; and chronological age, 118-119; and gain in height compared, 137-138; see also bones
bones, 87-88, 90, 190, 230-231, 232, 233, 264; see also bone age
Borer, K.T., 263, 264-265

Bowers, C., 143
bromocriptine, 102-103
Brown-Sequard, Charles, 48-49
Bush, Barbara, 27, 48
Bush, George, 27, 48
Byrne, Charles, 77

Caremark Homecare, 223-224
Carey, L.C., 245
Carney, Brent, 142, 143-164
carpal tunnel syndrome, 96
cartilage, cells, 68-69, 71, 113, 190; growth, 70, 90, 91
Cassoria, Fernando, 180-181, 191
children, appearance of GH-deficient, 138; GH-deficient, 15, 61-62, 63, 117-142, 143-164, 203, 239, 254; and GH therapy, 17, 118-120, 123, 128, 130-137, 143-164, 168-172; GH therapy for non-GH-deficient, 168-172; GH therapy for short, 168-172; growth rates of GH-deficient, 117; short, 17, 19-20, 168-172; symptoms of GH-deficient, 117
China, 37-38
Choh Hao Li, 59-60, 62, 217, 221

cholecystokin-pan-creozymin, 33
cholesterol, 16, 32
choriosomatomamma-tropin, 58
Christiansen, J. Sandahl, 228-229
Christy, James H., 89-91, 168
chromosomes, 51
chronological age, 127; and bone age, 118-119
Clemmons, David, 248
clonidine, 124
Coleman, Gary, 110
collagen, 231, 232, 256
corticosteroids, 32
corticotrophs, 65, 100
cortisol, 69, 114, 188
Cowart, Virginia, 252
Crawford, Albert, 50
cretinism, 27, 43, 111, 114, 187
Creutzfeldt-Jakob disease, 63
Crist, Douglas, 17, 254, 256
Cuneo, Ross, 227, 255
Cushing, Harvey, 56
Cushing's Disease, 114, 188

Darendeliler, F., 134, 135, 168, 178, 180, 189, 191
David, 75, 76
da Vinci, Leonardo, 41
de la Rosa, Nelson, 108
DES, 241

diabetes, 31, 36, 43, 49, 51, 90, 95, 99, 103, 168, 186, 242-243
dieting, 247-248, 249
Dinkas, 75
DNA, 62, 214
Doisy, Edward, 51
double-blind studies, 12, 169, 254
drug companies, 215-224; competition among, 221-222
Dupuy, Susan, 204, 205, 206
dwarfism, 27, 106-115; causes of, 114; Laron-type, 189-190; perceived, 174; psychological, 192-193; see also dwarfs
dwarfs, 79, 106-115, 120, 190-191; in culture, 106-107; in folk literature, 105-106; life expectancy of, 108; number of, in U.S., 113; shortest, 107-108; see also dwarfism

elderly, 9-15, 16; effects of GH on, 10-11, 13-14, 16, 249; GH-deficient, 19, 229-236, 247, 254
endocrine glands, 21-34, 95; diseases of, 26-27, 36; exocrine function of, 33-34
endocrinology, 21-34, history of, 35-51

epinephrine *see* adrenalin

epiphyses *see* growth plates

escherichia coli (e. coli), 62, 215-216, 219

estradiol, 235-237

estrogen, 32, 33, 38, 138, 175, 184, 235; deficiency and GH-deficiency, 235-238; replacement and GH, 238-240; replacement therapy, 49, 238-240; side effects of, replacement therapy, 239-240

Evans, Herbert, 57-58

exercise, 17, 66, 233; GH secretion and, 262-265

exocrine glands, 42

exophthalmus, 27

fat, 10, 16, 58, 69, 72, 233, 245, 254, 264

Federal Drug Administration (FDA), 15, 62, 63, 168, 177, 216, 219, 221, 223, 228, 257, 262

fertility, 240-241

Flynn, Margaret, 230

follicle stimulating hormone (FSH), 59, 65

Fost, Norman C., 166, 194-195, 196

Frasier, F. Douglas, 183, 195-196

Frye, Kim, 171, 203-204

Galen, 41

Galileo, 42

gamma globulin, 188

gastrin, 33

gastrointestinal tract, 71; disorders, 186, 194

Genentech, 168, 205, 215, 216-219, 220, 221, 222, 223-224, 253, 257

genetic disorders, 189-191, 201

Gertner, J.M., 180

giantism *see* gigantism

giants, 73-89, 108; familial, 75-77; pituitary, 75, 168

gigantism, 73-89; causes of, 86-89; cerebral, 87; diagnosis of, 80-81; in folk literature, 73-75; and GH, 75-78, 79-80, 88; in rats, 58

glucagon, 31, 124

glucocorticoids, 32

glucose suppression test, 101

goiter, 36, 38, 43

Goliath, 75, 76

gonadotrophs, 65, 95, 100, 138, 240-241

gonads, 21, 29, 228; rooster, 44; and secondary sex characteristics, 45-46

Graves' Disease, 27, 37, 47-48

Graves, Robert James, 47

Greece, 39, 40-41

growth, abnormal, 212; catch-down, 167; catch-up, 192; channels, 209, 211-212; charts, 81-83, 176-177, 198, 204, 205, 206, 211; delay, 182-184, 213; gender and, delay, 182-183; and GH production, 179-180; normal, rates, 117, 209; rates of GH-deficient children, 117, 174, 185; rates with combined therapies, 177; rates with GHRH therapy, 140; screenings, 204-208; spurt, 87, 191, 209, 213; spurt with GH, 133, 136; velocity with GH, 180-181, 183-184

growth disorders, 199-213; diagnosis of, 202-203; short stature as a, 211

growth hormone (GH), abuse of, 253, 255-256; administration of, 133-134, 136, 178-179, 185; aging and, deficiency, 230-233; and aging process, 10-11, 228-233; and amino acids, 18-19, 260-262; antibodies to, 219-220; athletes and use of, 251-165; ban on, 256; biosynthetic, 62, 63, 129, 131, 132, 134, 136, 167, 168, 173, 180, 215-222, 223, 224, 254, 255, 256; biosynthetic and pituitary compared, 133-134; black market, 257-258; blood levels, 70, 209-210, 246; body production of, 11-12, 78-79, 123, 124-128, 183, 188; continuous, therapy, 136-137; controversy over, therapy, 166-172; cost of, therapy, 15; and cretinism, 111; criteria for, therapy, 194-197, 222-223; dangers of, therapy, 123; deficiency and estrogen, 235-238; deficiency and psychological problems, 227-228; deficiency due to radiation therapy, 126, 141; -deficient adults, 226-229, 230-233; -deficient children, 15, 61-62, 63, 117-142, 143-164, 203, 239, 254; -deficient elderly, 19, 229-236, 247, 249, 254; definition of, deficiency, 62; diagnosis of, deficiency by gender, 129; diagnosis of, deficiency by race, 129-130; diagnosis of, deficiency in children, 120-128, 129-130; and dieting, 247-248, 249; discovery of, 58; distribution of, 223-224; doses of, 134, 135, 138, 178-179, 185; and dwarfism, 111; effects of, 10-11, 13-14, 16, 53-54, 58, 69, 70, 72, 225-226, 238, 263-264; effect of, on elderly, 10-11, 13-14, 16, 233-234, 249; and estradiol, 235-237; and exercise, 17, 66, 233, 262-265; fake, 253, 258; and fertility, 240-241; foreign-made, 252-253; and gigantism, 75-78, 79-80, 88; goals of, therapy, 130-133, 194; growth and, production, 179-180; growth spurts with, 133, 136; and healing, 241-244; illegal distribution of biosynthetic, 251-253; indirect action of, 67-69, 70; and insulin, 69-70; insurance for, therapy, 176-177, 178; intermittent, therapy, 136-137; iodinated, 67; isolation of, 59-61; and lack of food, 246-247; long-term effects of, therapy, 19, 233-234; manufacturing biosynthetic, 215-217; measurements of, effect, 14; molecular weight of, 54; molecule, 61; and muscle-building, 253-256; and muscle/fat ratios, 226-229; and nitrogen balance, 247; origin of ex-

cess, 100-101; orphan drug status of biosynthetic, 217, 218, 219, 220-221; and oxandrolone, 177-178; pituitary, 55-56, 63, 110, 120, 131, 134, 218, 219, 222; and pituitary gland, 55-56, 75-78, 79-80, 88, 89, 90, 92-99, 110, 120, 141, 218; placental, 120; problems of excessive, 73-103, 233, 260; and protein supplements, 258-262; psychological uses for, 181; receptors, 67, 70, 71, 77, 86, 115, 264; -related disorders, 73-103; release patterns, 65-66, 70-72, 125; "releasers," 18-19; response to, therapy, 134-135; rhesus monkey, 54, 61; secretion, 12, 123-124, 135, 166, 175-176, 183, 210, 226, 229, 234, 235-238, 239, 245, 248, 256, 262-265; secretion of, during puberty, 137; side effects of, therapy, 138-140, 181, 234; and skeletal growth, 53, 71; and stress, 66, 244-247; structure of, 54; as substitute for anabolic steroids, 252, 256; supraphysiological levels of, 255, 256; and surgery, 245,

247, 249; surges of, 65-66, 210, 245-246, 260-261; tests of, production, 123, 124-128, 137, 166, 175, 176, 180, 183, 258; therapy, 9-15, 16, 19, 35, 49, 61, 118-120, 123, 128, 130-137, 143-164, 166-172, 223, 225, 228-229, 251-265; therapy for treatment of other diseases, 170, 171, 172-176; therapy for non-, -deficient children, 168-172; therapy for other growth disorders, 178-193, 201-203; therapy for short children, 168-172, 222-223; therapy for treatment of Turner Syndrome, 170, 171, 172-178, 201-203; treatment for diabetes, 242-243; use of, on elderly, 9-15, 69, 233-234, 249-250; in vitro, 63; in vivo, 63

growth hormone release inhibiting hormone (GH-IH), 64, 70, 71, 103

growth hormone releasing hormone (GHRH), 64, 65, 70-71, 100, 140-142, 239; administration of, 141-142; biosynthetic, 140; deficiency, 140-141; therapy, 140-142

growth hormone releasing peptide (GHRP), 142

growth plates, 74, 78, 87, 88, 90, 97, 98, 112, 118, 121, 139, 182, 186, 189, 202, 209, 225

Gynex, 177-178

hand bones, 74

Harvey, William, 42

Hashimoto's Disease, 187

heart, 25-26, 95, 123

height, gain in, and bone age compared, 137-138; and growth spurts, 83; mid-parental average, 131-132; normal, for boys, 81-82

Heisler, Lorenz, 43

Herodotus, 75

Hintz, Raymond, 227, 255

Hippocrates, 39

histamine, 30

Ho, K.Y., 235-236, 238

Hooke, Robert, 42

hormone releasing factors, 28

hormone replacement therapy, 33, 49, 102; ancient, 37-38

Hormone Research Laboratory, 59

hormones, adrenal cortex, 32-33, 69, 228; adrenal medulla, 31-32; circulation of, 44-46; disorders,

187-189; gastrointestinal, 33; heart, 33; hypothalamus, 29, 71; lung, 33; luteinizing, 59; milk-making, 28, 38, 58, 65, 95-96; ovarian, 32, 33, 51; pancreatic islands, 31; pineal, 30-31; pituitary, 57, 58, 59, 60, 61, 64, 65, 100, 240-241; placental, 33; and puberty, 191; sex, 32, 38, 87, 228, 235; testes, 32; thymic, 31; thyroid, 27, 30, 87, 111, 118, 121, 137, 139, 228; trophic, 28, 29, 95, 102; *see also* growth hormone; specific hormones

Horner family, 170-171

Human Growth Foundation, 203, 204, 205, 208

Humatrope, 136, 218-219, 220, 224, 243

humors, 39-40, 42, 55

Hunter, John, 46, 77

Hunt, Linda, 110-112

Hyman, Flo, 86

hypochondroplasia, 113, 190-191

hypoglycemia test, 125-126

hypothalamus, 21, 25, 28, 29, 39, 43, 63, 64-65, 71, 72, 140, 190, 240, 256; diseases, 141; feedback system, 70-72, 190, 264; hormones, 29, 71

immune system, 31, 226, 227, 232

impotence, 95

inhibiting factors, 28

Institute of Experimental Biology, 58, 59

insulin, 31, 70, 87, 90, 124, 243; and diabetes, 49; and GH, 69-70; resistance, 123, 139

insulinlike growth factor II, 87

insurance companies, 171, 176-177, 178

intersex, 36

intrauterine growth retardation (IUGR), 184-186

iodine, 30, 38, 50

Iodogen, 67

Jacobson, Bert, 255, 256, 260

Job, Jean-Claude, 139

Jorgensen, J.O.L., 16

Joyner, Florence Griffith, 252

Kaplan, Pam, 204, 205, 207, 208

Kessler, David, 223

kidney, 95, 232, 233; diseases, 186-187

Klinefelter Syndrome, 87

Koehler, Don, 79

kypho-scoliosis, 80; *see also* scoliosis

lactogens, 58

lactotrophs, 65, 100

Lantos, John, 181

Laron, Zvi, 189-190

lean body mass, 10, 16, 230, 264

Leeuwenhock, 42

Leggett, Donald, 257

Lemon, Peter, 259

leukemia, 139, 141

levodopa (L. dopa), 124, 125; test, 125

Lifshitz, Fima, 193

Lincoln, Abraham, 86-87, 109

Linder, Barbara, 180-181, 188, 191

Lilly, Eli and Company, 218-219, 220, 221, 243, 251, 253, 257

Lippe, Barbara, 195-196

Little People of America, 113-114

liver, 67, 68, 71, 72, 95, 232, 233, 239-240

lung tumors, 100

luteinizing hormone (LH), 59, 65

lymph system, 43

lysine, 258, 260-261

Magrath, Cornelius, 77

malnutrition, 191-192, 193, 264

Manasco, Penelope, 189

Manson, James, 244

Marfan Syndrome, 86-87

Mark, Leonard, 99-100

Martha, P.M., 125

McGauley, G.A., 228

Medvei, Victor, 36, 44, 48, 49, 75, 76, 77, 107

melatonin, 30

menopause, 235, 236, 238, 239

menstruation, 95

met-GH *see* somatrem

methionine, 218, 219

midget, 114

mineralocorticoids, 32

Minkowski, Oscar, 51

Mirbeck, Sieur, 77-78

Mojane, Gabriele, 79

Murray, George, 49

muscle, 245; atrophy of, 14; GH and, -building, 253-255; mass, 227, 230, 233, 248; strength, 227, 230, 233; versus performance, 255-256

Musters, Pauline, 107

Myllyrinne, Vaino, 79

myxedema, 27, 49

Nagraj, Hoshote, 11

National Center for Health Statistics (NCHS) growth charts, 81-83, 198, 204, 205, 206, 211

National Cooperative

Growth Study (NCGS), 224

norepinephrine, 31-32, 38

obesity, 247-248, 249
ocreotide, 103
Oliver, George, 49-50
organotherapy, 37, 48-49
Oriti, Marco, 170
ornithine, 18-19, 124, 258, 260, 261
Orphan Drug Act of 1983, 217, 218, 219, 220-221
osteoporosis, 231, 239
ovaries, 23, 32, 33, 38, 239, 240; cysts on, 139; hormones, 32, 33, 51
ovulation, 43, 240, 241; cessation of, 95
Oxandrin, 178
oxandrolone, 177-178
oxytocin, 29

pancreas, 23, 31, 43, 51, 70, 87, 95; diseases, 87, 102; tumors, 64, 102
pancreatic islands, 23, 31, 51; hormones, 31; tumors, 100
parathyroid gland, 23, 30, 51; hormones, 30-31
parathyroid hormone (PTH), 30
Parks, John S., 78, 122, 166, 169, 183, 191, 192, 211, 212, 213

pediatricians, 202-203
peptides, 61
Pfaffle, Roland, 122
Phillips, Calvin, 108
pineal gland, 23, 30-31; hormones, 30-31
pituitary gland, 21, 23, 28-29, 41, 43, 61, 65, 71, 125, 140, 190, 228, 240, 256, 264; anterior, hormones, 57, 58, 59, 60, 61, 100; anterior lobe, 29-30, 56, 57, 58, 64, 65, 75, 100; diseases, 29, 43, 56, 57, 69, 141; and excess GH production, 75-78, 79-80, 88, 89, 90, 92-99, 100-101; and GH, 55-56, 75-78, 79-80, 88-89, 90, 92-99, 110, 120, 141; hormones, 57, 58, 59, 60, 61, 64, 65, 95, 100; hyperactive, 57, 76, 100, 101; hypoactive, 57, 69, 101, 102, 121, 140, 170, 213, 241; location of, 55-56; role of, in acromegaly, 99-100; role of, in growth, 57; surgery, 91-92, 102; treatment for, tumors, 102; tumors, 43, 56, 75, 77, 88, 89, 90, 92, 93, 94, 95, 96, 98, 99, 100-101
placenta, 33, 54
Pliny the Elder, 37, 114
polytomography, 101
progesterone, 32-33

prolactin, 28, 38, 58, 65, 95-96, 100, 102-103

prolactin inhibiting factors (PIF), 28

prostaglandins, 33

Protropin, 129, 136, 168, 218, 220, 222, 223; sales, 222, 223-224

proteins, 258-262; complete, 259, 260; RDA of, 259; supplements, 258-262; vegetable, 259

provocation tests, 176, 180, 183

puberty, 88, 127, 135, 137-138, 182, 193, 209, 210, 226, 235; delayed, 138, 166, 182-184, 264; and growth, 81-84, 87-88, 209, 210, 211-212, 214; and hormones, 191; inducing, 175; precocious, 87-88, 188-189, 191, 213; sex hormones and 184

pygmies, 114-115

Pythagoras, 39-40

Raben, Maurice S., 61

radioimmunoassay (RIA), 126-127

radio receptor assay, 67

Rainer, Adam, 108

Rasmussen, Lars, 243

receptors, 67, 70, 71, 77, 86, 115, 264

Reiter, E.O., 125

Riddle, Oscar, 58

Rogan, John William, 79

Romans, 40-41

Rosenfeld, R.G., 174

Rose, Susan, 123-124, 127, 128

Rudman, Daniel, 10, 180, 225-226, 229, 230, 231, 232, 238

Rudman study, 9-15, 16, 19, 69, 233-234, 249, 254

Salk Institute, 64

Salomon, Franco, 16

Sanders, David, 184-185

Schaefer, Edward, 49-50, 56

scoliosis, 86, 96; see also kypho-scoliosis

Searle, G.D. Company, 177-178

secretin, 33

sella turcica, 55, 77, 92, 99, 101

sensory organs, 21, 25

serotonin, 30

sex hormones, 32, 38, 87, 228, 235

sex steroids, 32, 118

short stature, 166, 185, 196, 223; criteria for, 210-213; as a disorder, 211; famil-ial, 179-181, 199-200, 207, 212-213; idiopathic, 194

skeleton, deformities, 96; dysplasia, 190; growth, 53, 71, 209 skin, 231-232; atrophy of, 14; thickness of, 231-232

Slavin, Joanne, 260

SmC/IGF-I, 68-69, 71, 72, 180, 187, 190, 227, 239, 240, 248, 254, 255, 264; blood levels, 71

Smith, Philip, 58

somatomedin A, 68

somatomedin B, 68

somatomedin C see SmC/IGF-I

somatostatin see GH-IH

somatotrophs, 65, 100

somatotropin see growth hormone

Soto's Syndrome, 87

somatrem, 63, 217-218

Spallanzani, Lazzaro, 43-44

sperm, 42, 43

spleen, 95, 232, 233

spontaneous testing, 123, 124, 126-128; versus stimulation testing, 126-128

Stanhope, R., 185

stimulation testing, 123, 124-125, 126-128, 137, 166, 175, 195; versus spontaneous testing, 126-128

Stratton, Charles see Thumb, Tom

stress, 66, 244-247

sulfation factor, 68

systemic disease, 186-187

tall stature, familial, 83-86

Tanaka, Toshiaki, 175, 176

Tanner, J.M., 130, 131-132, 168-170

teeth, movement of, 92-93

testes, 23, 32, 33-34, 40; hormones, 32, 33-34; transplants, in animals, 45-46

testosterone, 32, 33, 138, 184, 236

Thorner, Michael, 140, 141, 235-236, 238, 239

Thumb, Tom, 108-110

thymin, 31

thymosin, 31

thymus, 23, 31, 43, hormones, 31

thyroid gland, 21, 23, 41, 43, 50, 95, 187, 213, 228; diseases of, 27, 36, 38, 47-48; hormones, 28, 30, 87, 111, 118, 121; hypoactive, 27, 136, 139, 187-188, 208, 213; hyperactive, 27, 87; parrot, 46

thyroid stimulating hormone (TSH), 28

thyroid-stimulating-hormone releasing hormone (TRH), 28

thyrotrophin, 65

thyrotrophin releasing hormone, 101

thyrotrophs, 65, 100

thyroxin, 29, 30, 114, 121, 136, 187, 188

transphenoidal microsur-
gery, 91-92, 102
triiodothyronine, 30
Turner Syndrome, 172-178,
189, 193, 195, 196, 201,
208, 213; and GH secre-
tion, 175-176; symptoms
of, 172-173

Underwood, Louis, 248
urine therapy, 37-38

Vance, Mary Lee, 15
Vanderschueren-
Lodeweyckx, M., 128
Van Wyk, Judson J., 69
vasopressin, 29
Vesalius, Andreas, 41
von Baer, Carl, 51

von Mering, Joseph, 51

Waago, Harald, 242-243
Wadlaw, Robert, 78-79
Ward, John, 96
Watusis, 75
Werth, Barry, 221-222
Wilmore, Douglas, 244
Wit, J.M., 121-122

XYY Chromosome Syn-
drome 87

Yamashiro, Donald, 61

Zaccheus, 106-107
Zeng Jinlian, 78